OREGON
MAP KEY

Other titles in this series

THE BEST IN TENT CAMPING

A GUIDE FOR CAR CAMPERS WHO HATE RVs,
CONCRETE SLABS, AND LOUD PORTABLE STEREOS

OREGON

SECOND EDITION

Jeanne Louise Pyle
revised by Paul Gerald

MENASHA RIDGE PRESS
BIRMINGHAM, ALABAMA

*This book is gratefully dedicated to everybody who works
so hard to get the campgrounds ready for us and takes care of them
after we go.*

Copyright © 2009 by Jeanne Louise Pyle and Paul Gerald

All rights reserved

Printed in the United States of America

Published by Menasha Ridge Press

Distributed by Publishers Group West

Second edition, first printing

Library of Congress Cataloging-in-Publication Data

Pyle, Jeanne L., 1954–
   The best in tent camping, Oregon : a guide for car campers who hate RVs, concrete slabs,
   and loud portable stereos / Jeanne Louise Pyle ; revised by Paul Gerald. — 2nd ed.
      p. cm.
   Includes bibliographical references and index.
   ISBN-13: 978-0-89732-706-0 (alk. paper)
   ISBN-10: 0-89732-706-3 (alk. paper)
      1. Camping—Oregon—Guidebooks. 2. Camp sites, facilities, etc.—Oregon—Guidebooks.
   3. Oregon—Guidebooks. I. Gerald, Paul. II. Title.
   GV191.42.O7P95 2009
   796.5409795--dc22
                                          2009019617

Cover and text design by Ian Szymkowiak, Palace Press International, Inc.

Cover photo by Danita Delimont / Alamy

Maps by Steve Jones

Menasha Ridge Press

P.O. Box 43673

Birmingham, Alabama 35243

www.menasharidge.com

TABLE OF CONTENTS

ACKNOWLEDGMENTS

This book came about with the assistance of numerous people who provided information, guidance, feedback, insights, and most importantly, encouragement.
Specifically, we'd like to thank:

All of the National Forest Service, Bureau of Land Management, and individual park staff who provided accurate information, campground layouts, and other vital information to make these entries as exact as possible. They often had to dig deep and they came up with exactly what I needed when I needed it. These include—and we hope we got all the names—Jennifer McDonald, Bob Henning, Erik Taylor, Barb Smith, Traci Meredith, Mike Hall, Nancy Rudger, Rob Bundy, Carole Picard, Janel Lacey, Fred McDonald, Shannon Winegar, Sandy Loop, Tom Mottl, Jerry Johnson, Debra Drake, Dwight Johnson, David Grimes, Cindy Pack, Nicole Malandri, Sheri Cameron, Nicole Malandri, John Zapell, and Jo and Don of Pampering Campers.

Also thanks to Duane Graham at Summer Lake Hot Springs for advice, charm, and hot water, and to Rich and Val Allyn of Depoe Bay, Oregon, who were the delightful camp hosts at Tumalo State Park in Bend and who took time from their busy schedules to help out with the chapter on Canal Creek Campground.

PREFACE

Fifty campgrounds for just one state. Fifty seems like a big number, doesn't it? What are the odds that one person—you, for example—will ever camp in all 50 places described in this book?

Well, you should know that it took two of us just to visit and describe these 50 places. Jeanne Louise Pyle created the first edition of this book for its 2004 publication, and in 2008, Menasha Ridge Press asked me to revise it. They said something like "get some new ones in there and make sure the other ones are still up to date."

No worries, right? Just send the chapters to some very helpful government folks, then drive around and find "some new ones." It's just one state, right?

Well, not really. The idea that Silver Falls, the Hart Mountain Refuge, and Camp Blanco share even a continent, much less a state, with the streetcars and high rises of Portland is a bit mind-boggling. And we Portlanders, it must be said, have a highly skewed idea of our state. We cut it into "western" and "eastern," thus lumping Prineville, the Wallowas, Steens Mountain, and Lakeview into some vague "other" place that we are only marginally aware of.

No matter where you live, but especially if you live in Portland or the Willamette Valley, it's my sincere hope that you'll use this book as a guide to exploring Oregon. Don't say, "Well, next time we get out east, we should check out some of these campsites." Instead, say, "Let's go out to Steens Mountain this year and camp there." Or say, "I've always heard the Blue Mountains are nice, so let's pack up the camping gear and check 'em out." Or, even better, find someplace in here you've never even heard of and go see it. I bet there are some within a couple hours of your house.

For me, updating Jeanne's fantastic work was a constant stream of "discoveries." The fact I lived in Portland 13 years before I went to the top of the Steens is somewhat embarrassing. I had never really explored the Elkhorn Mountains, only passed through the Gearhardt Mountain area, and never seen the antelope in the wide-open spaces of the Hart Mountain refuge.

Likewise, as many times as I had hiked Eagle Creek, just 45 minutes from where I live, I'd never seen the quaint and historic campground there. I had also never camped at Oxbow Regional Park in my own city's suburbs; and when I did, I was able to sit on a riverbank and watch spawning salmon thrash around in the rapids with a bald eagle overhead and fall colors all around. I'd never been to Waldo Lake but now plan to spend a week there sometime. And I thought I had known peace in the Three Sisters until I saw the campsites around Scott Lake.

It's those moments of discovery and serenity that we're looking for when we pitch our tent. And those moments, at least in our plans, don't include the sound of a buzzing generator or "boom box." So when evaluating campsites for this book, we have tried to take into account all the factors one would want in a place to lay one's head: peace, tranquility, some measure of privacy balanced with convenience, and a nice view.

The truth is, however, that when traveling to any of these campsites, you'll drive past plenty of others that could have made the book. In fact, part of my standard conversation with BLM and Forest Service employees always included me saying, "I know I should check out the other five places you're telling me about in your area, but I've only got 50 for the whole state!"

So while we offer this book as an invitation to explore our beautiful state, we also hope it won't limit you. If you see a tree-lined gravel road and a sign saying, "Campground, 8 miles," go check it out! Neither Jeanne nor I have been to every place in the state, but we've been to every place in this book, and a heck of a lot of others. By all means, go find your own little treasures, and if you're willing to share your discoveries, drop us a line.

Meanwhile, may the book you're holding lead you, your friends, and your family to many wonderful times in Oregon. It's a big, beautiful state—actually several states in one it seems—and exploring it for this book has been a fine and humbling experience

—Paul Gerald

INTRODUCTION

From rocky coastlines to alpine meadows to sagebrush deserts, Oregon is a place of unparalleled beauty and diversity. Extremes of climate, terrain, and vegetation can be experienced in a single day's outing. The campgrounds included in this book are representative of the variety that makes Oregon such a prized destination for those who seek outstanding outdoor adventures.

And for those who value an experience that is long on solitude, serenity, and space, be aware that you may have to seek adventure farther afield than most. To escape the crowds, you must drive farther, climb higher, and plan more creatively. Although Oregon ranks third behind Alaska and Washington in designated wilderness acreage, it still constitutes only a little more than three percent of the state's total amount of land. More and more people flock beyond city limits to these scenic natural splendors, pushing the state's wilderness boundaries to capacity.

Encountering RVs in the most unlikely of places, one has to wonder if it isn't more comforting to think of wilderness as a state of mind rather than an actual place. For some tent campers, it is satisfaction enough just to pitch a tent alongside several hundred others in midsummer at the busy, nearby state park. For others, simply being able to drive to the campground eliminates it from consideration. If your sentiment lies somewhere between these two extremes, you should find the offerings in this book appealing.

Naturally, there are factors besides crowds that impact every camping trip, from a last minute trip to the outskirts of town to a backcountry outing planned months in advance. Here is some information that will prove useful, whether you are a first-time camper in Oregon or a veteran (you can always use a few reminders).

GEOGRAPHIC REGIONS

For a traveler, the most obvious distinction within Oregon is the difference in climate, terrain, and, to some degree, lifestyle between the western and eastern regions of the state. The rugged coast and the Cascade mountains, which run north–south through the state, are generally considered Western Oregon, while Eastern Oregon (larger and sparsely populated) includes vast stretches of arid land. For ease in planning your trip, however, we have further grouped campgrounds into six regions, dividing those along the coast into northern and southern groups, dividing those in the Cascades (home to a prepoderance of Oregon's campgrounds) into northern, central, and southern groups, and presenting the scattered offerings of Eastern Oregon in a single group. If you intend, for example, to make Crater Lake the primary destination for your camping trip, you will first want to review campgrounds in the Southern Cascades.

THE OVERVIEW MAP AND OVERVIEW-MAP KEY

Use the overview map on the inside front cover to assess the exact location of each campground. The campground's number appears not only on the overview map but also on the map key facing the overview map, in the table of contents, and on the profile's first page.

The book is organized by region, as indicated in the table of contents. A map legend that details the symbols found on the campground layout maps appears on the inside back cover.

CAMPGROUND-LAYOUT MAPS

Each profile contains a detailed campground-layout map that provides an overhead look at campground sites, internal roads, facilities, and other key items. Each campground entrance's GPS coordinates are included with each profile.

GPS CAMPGROUND-ENTRANCE COORDINATES

Readers can easily access all campgrounds in this book by using the directions given and the overview map, which shows at least one major road leading into the area. But for those who enjoy using the latest GPS technology to navigate, the necessary data has been provided. This book includes the GPS coordinates for each campground. For readers who own a GPS unit, whether handheld or onboard a vehicle, the Universal Transverse Mercator (UTM) coordinates provided with each campground description may be entered into the GPS unit. Just make sure your GPS unit is set to navigate using the UTM system in conjunction with WGS84 datum.

UTM COORDINATES: ZONE, EASTING, AND NORTHING

Within the UTM coordinates box within each campground description, there are three numbers labeled zone, easting, and northing. Here is an example from Cascadia State Park Campground:

> UTM Zone (WGS84)   10T
> Easting   0541324
> Northing   4916134

The zone number (10) refers to one of the 60 longitudinal zones (vertical) of a map using the UTM projection. Each zone is 6° wide. The zone letter (T) refers to one of the 20 latitudinal zones (horizontal) that span from 80° South to 84° North. The easting number (0541324) references in meters how far east the point is from the zero value for eastings, which runs north-south through Greenwich, England. Increasing easting coordinates on a topo map or on your GPS screen indicate you are moving east; decreasing easting coordinates indicate you are moving west. Since lines of longitude converge at the poles, they are not parallel as lines of latitude are. This means that the distance between Full Easting Coordinates is 1,000 meters near the equator but becomes smaller as you travel farther north or south; the difference is small enough to be ignored, but only until you reach the polar regions.

In the Northern Hemisphere, the northing number (4916134) references in meters how far you are from the equator. Above the equator, northing coordinates increase by

1,000 meters between each parallel line of latitude (east-west lines). On a topo map or GPS receiver, increasing northing numbers indicate you are traveling north.

In the Southern Hemisphere, the northing number references how far you are from a latitude line that is 10 million meters south of the equator. Below the equator, northing coordinates decrease by 1,000 meters between each line of latitude. On a topo map, decreasing northing coordinates indicate you are traveling south.

WEATHER

Prevailing conditions year-round (with a few exceptions) in western Oregon are mild and damp. Not so much rain, as a healthy supply of gray clouds and mist. Areas like the Willamette Valley on the eastern flanks of the Coast Range can get quite hot and steamy, but a short drive up and over the range to the coastal areas and you'll be reaching for the fleece as the inversion effect creates fog banks and cool breezes. Late summer and early fall are the most dependable seasons for lovely stints of dry, sunny, warm days just about anywhere in western Oregon.

In eastern Oregon, conditions are desert-like, with hot and dry summers. Severe thunderstorms can be the biggest threat to outdoor activity and, in turn, can spark wildfires and flash floods. At higher elevations on both western and eastern mountain slopes, snow is common, even in midsummer. Sudden changes in weather conditions are always a consideration, so pack accordingly.

ROAD CONDITIONS AND DIRECTIONS

Many of the campgrounds in this book are reached by minimally maintained access roads. Since we were looking for spots that are somewhat off the beaten path (and away from the most-traveled routes for those dreaded RVs), access roads can be rougher than you might expect. Inquire about current road conditions before venturing too far if you are unsure of what you may encounter and be sure that you have a current road atlas with you.

The maps in this book are designed to help orient you, nothing more. Although we've provided directions at the end of each entry, you'll still need detailed maps to get in and out of most of the campgrounds. The local and district offices that oversee most of these campgrounds are the best source for detailed maps (see Appendix B for more information on these agencies).

Standardized road designations appear throughout the text in accordance with the following examples: I-5 for Interstate 5, US 101 for U.S. Highway 101, OR 58 for Oregon Highway 58, SR 205 for State Road 205, CR 40 for County Road 40, and FS 15 for Forest Service Road 15.

RESTRICTIONS

Increased visitation to natural areas usually means more restrictions. State and federal agencies manage most of the campgrounds in this book. Check with the proper authorities for current regulations on recreational activities, such as permits for day-use parking, backcountry travel, hunting and fishing, mountain bikes in designated areas, etc. We have included some restrictions in the Key Information sections of each campground description, but because restrictions can change, you still need to check before you go. Be aware that many national forest and State Park parking areas now require day-use fees or annual passes. Passes can be purchased at any forest service office or ranger station, and at numerous campgrounds and outdoor retailer outlets.

FIRES

Campfire regulations are subject to seasonal conditions. Usually there are signs posted at campgrounds or ranger district offices. Please be sure you are aware of the current situation and NEVER make a campfire anywhere other than in existing fire pits at developed sites. Never, ever toss a match or cigarette idly in the brush or alongside the road. It's not only littering, it can also trigger the incineration of that beautiful forest you were just admiring.

WATER

Many of the campgrounds in this book are remote enough that piped water is not available. No matter how remote you may think you are, though, don't risk drinking straight from mountain streams, creeks, and lakes. Oregon has some of the purest natural waters in the world, but it is not immune to that nasty parasite called Giardia lamblia, which causes horrific stomach cramps and long-term diarrhea. If you don't have drinking water or purification tablets with you, boil any untreated water for at least five minutes. This will seem like a hassle if you're dry as a bone at the end of a long day of activity, but believe me, the agony you will avoid makes it worth the wait.

THE RATING SYSTEM

Within the scope of the campground criteria for this book—accessible by car, scenic, and as close to a wilderness setting as possible—each campground offers its own characteristics. The best way to deal with these varying attributes was to devise a rating system that highlights each campground's best features. On our five-star ranking system, five is the highest rating and one is the lowest. So if you're looking for a campground that is scenic and achingly quiet, look for five stars in the Beauty and Quiet categories. If you're more interested in a campground that has excellent security and cavernous campsites, look for five stars in the Spaciousness and Security categories. Keep in mind that these ratings are based somewhat on the subjective views of the authors.

BEAUTY   If this category needs explanation at all, it is simply to say that the true beauty of a campground is not always what you can see but what you can't see. Or hear. Like a freeway. Or motorboats. Or a rifle range. An equally important factor is the condition of the campground itself—and to what extent it has been left in its natural state. Beauty, of course, also takes into consideration any fabulous views of mountains, waterfalls, or other natural phenomena.

SITE PRIVACY   No one who enjoys the simplicity of tent camping wants to be walled in on all sides by RVs the size of tractor trailers. This category goes hand in hand with the previous one, because in part a campsite's beauty relies on the privacy of its surroundings. If you've ever crawled out of your tent to embrace a stunning summer morning in your skivvies and found several pairs of curious eyes staring at you from the neighbor's picture window, you know what we mean. We look for campsites that are graciously spaced with lots of heavy foliage in between. You can often find more private sites by driving a little deeper into the campground complex.

SPACIOUSNESS   Size isn't a big deal to us, as long as there's room to park the car off the main campground road, enough space to pitch a two- or four-man tent in a reasonably flat and dry spot, a picnic table, and a fire pit safely away from the tenting area. At many campgrounds, site spaciousness is sacrificed for site privacy and vice versa. Sometimes you get extremely lucky and have both. Don't be greedy.

QUIET   Again, this category coincides with the beauty field. When I go camping, I want to hear the sounds of nature. You know, birds chirping, the wind sighing, a surf crashing, a brook babbling. Call me crazy . . . it's not always possible to control the noise volume of your fellow campers, so the closer you can get to natural sounds that can drown them out, the better. Actually, when you have a chance to listen to the quiet of nature, you'll find that it is really rather noisy. But what a lovely cacophony!

SECURITY   Quite a few of the campgrounds in this book are in remote and primitive places without on-site security patrols. In essence, you're on your own. Common sense is a great asset in these cases. Don't leave expensive outdoor gear or valuable camera equipment lying around your campsite—or even within view inside your car. If you are at a hosted site, you may feel more comfortable leaving any valuables with the host (if they're willing). Or let them know when you'll be gone for an extended period so they can keep an eye on your things. Unfortunately, even in lightly camped areas, vandalism is a common camping problem. In many places, wild animals can do as much damage as a human being. If you leave food inside your tent or around the campsite, don't be surprised if things look slightly ransacked when you return. The most frequent visitors to food-strewn campsites are birds, squirrels, chipmunks, deer, and bears.

CLEANLINESS   By and large, all the campgrounds in this book rank highly in this category. Oregon campgrounds are some of the cleanest and tidiest around; the only time they tend to fall a bit short of expectation is on busy summer weekends. This is usually only the case for larger, more developed compounds. In more remote areas, the level of cleanliness is most often dependent on the good habits of campers themselves. Keep that in mind wherever you camp. If the sign says, "Pack it in, pack it out," do as you're told. You can dump your garbage at the first gas station. DON'T expect someone to pick up after you at the campsite.

INSECT CONTROL   Spraying for bugs is not a regular practice in Oregon campgrounds. If the campground is situated on a lake (particularly at higher elevations), you can almost bet that mosquitoes will be a nuisance in midsummer. Even if the campground has earned a high insect control rating, it's always a good idea to have a reliable repellent in your cache of camping essentials. Everyone reacts to (and is affected by) the presence of bugs differently. The most common critters that cause problems are mosquitoes, no-see-ums, deer flies, sand fleas, and ticks.

FIRST-AID KIT

A useful first-aid kit may contain more items than you might think necessary. These are just the basics. Prepackaged kits in waterproof bags (Atwater Carey and Adventure Medical make them) are available. As a preventive measure, take along sunscreen and insect repellent. Even though quite a few items are listed here, they pack down into a small space:

Ace bandages or Spenco joint wraps

Adhesive bandages, such as Band-Aids

Antibiotic ointment (Neosporin or the generic equivalent)

Antiseptic or disinfectant, such as Betadine or hydrogen peroxide

Aspirin or acetaminophen

Benadryl or the generic equivalent, diphenhydramine (in case of allergic reactions)

Butterfly-closure bandages

Comb and tweezers (for removing stray cactus needles from your skin)

Emergency poncho

Epinephrine in a prefilled syringe (for people known to have severe allergic reactions to such things as bee stings)

Gauze (one roll)

Gauze compress pads (six 4- x 4-inch pads)

LED flashlight or headlamp

Matches or pocket lighter

Mirror for signaling passing aircraft

Moleskin/Spenco Second Skin

Pocketknife or multipurpose tool

Waterproof first-aid tape

Whistle (it's more effective in signaling rescuers than your voice)

CHANGES

While campgrounds are less prone to change than big-time tourist attractions, they are nevertheless subject to agency budgets, upgrades and dilapidation, and even natural disasters. With that in mind, it's a good idea to call ahead for the most updated report on the campground you've selected. We appreciate being told about any notable changes that you come across while using this book and welcome all reader input, including suggestions for potential entries for future editions. Send them to the author care of Menasha Ridge Press at the address provided on the copyright page.

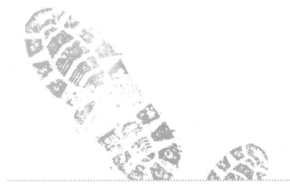

CENTRAL **CASCADES**

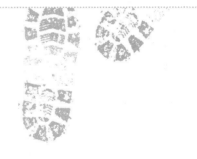

DRIVING EAST ON US 20 out of Sweet Home, you first pass Foster Lake, a large and decidedly un-scenic reservoir created by the Army Corps of Engineers. Then the road gets a little curvy, the trees get taller and thicker, and you can feel the draw of the high country. You start to speed up, dreaming of what's to come, and . . . what was that? Some kind of a park or something?

Yes, that sign on the left said Cascadia State Park, and it is one of the unknown gems of the Oregon State Park system. It doesn't have the magical attractions of Silver Falls (page 103) or the mountain scenery of Tumalo (page 32), and even the location wouldn't seem to inspire. But drive down that short access road, and you're in a little cove of peace and tranquility that most people speed right on past.

Cascadia actually has a manicured feel to it, like somebody designed it to be peaceful and inviting. That's because it's a former resort, built to entice visitors to Soda Creek. In the early 20th Century, the mineral-filled waters brought enough people to support a large hotel called the Geisendorfer, which had tennis courts, a garden, and a croquet course. I didn't know all this when I camped at Cascadia, but when I was in the big, mowed meadow by the group camping area, tossing a Frisbee barefoot in the summer sun, thinking that later I'd follow a trail down to the river for a swim and some fishing, it did occur to me that somebody did a good job putting this place together.

Cascadia relaxes under tall firs and hemlocks. It's bathed in fall colors from maples. It's awash in wildflowers in spring and early summer. Somehow, even when it's full, it's nice and quiet. The camp host once told me, "We're just a quiet little family park."

> *An island of tranquility between civilization and forested mountains, Cascadia is one of the gems of Oregon's state parks.*

RATINGS

Beauty: ☆ ☆ ☆ ☆
Privacy: ☆ ☆ ☆
Spaciousness: ☆ ☆ ☆
Quiet: ☆ ☆ ☆ ☆ ☆
Security: ☆ ☆ ☆ ☆
Cleanliness: ☆ ☆ ☆ ☆ ☆
Insect Control: ☆ ☆ ☆

KEY INFORMATION

ADDRESS: Cascadia State Park
P.O. Box 736
Cascadia, OR 97329

OPERATED BY: Oregon State Parks

INFORMATION: (541) 367-6021, (800) 551-6949, www.oregon stateparks.org

OPEN: May 1–September 30

SITES: 25

EACH SITE: Picnic tables, fire rings

ASSIGNMENT: First come, first served; no reservations

REGISTRATION: With host

FACILITIES: Piped water, day-use area, picnic sites with fireplaces and drinking fountains, two group sites ($61 per night) with covered kitchen area and electricity, reserved for a $6 fee through Reservations Northwest at (800) 452-5687

PARKING: At sites

FEE: $14; $5 per extra vehicle

ELEVATION: 850 feet

RESTRICTIONS: *Pets:* On leash only
Fires: In fire pits only
Alcohol: Permitted
Vehicles: RVs and trailers up to 35 feet

I once heard someone say of Cascadia, "There's nothing there, really, but campsites and forest and some trails and the river." To which I say, exactly!

The South Santiam River is, in these parts, a little wonder of Cascade scenery. It isn't awesome by any means, though in late spring I'm sure there's a ton of water in it. By late summer it's basically a series of deep, clear pools surrounded by cliffs and beautiful rock formations, separated by tiny rapids and waterfalls—perfect, in other words, for swimming or skipping around on the rocks, or even some fishing. You'll be lucky to catch anything bigger than 6 inches; the real fishing is below Foster Dam, where overlapping runs of Chinook salmon and steelhead bring folks from all over.

Other than fishing, swimming and lounging, Cascadia has two hiking trails that start right in the park: the River Trail runs one mile along the South Santiam, with several side trails leading down to the river. The Soda Falls Trail is a bit tougher, gaining 500 feet in less than a mile to 150-foot Lower Soda Creek Falls.

Again, the "real" hiking, if that's what you're into, is not at Cascadia; it's all over the place, just up US 20. Highlights include two former lookout sites, one atop a huge pillar called Rooster Rock (reached by a steep 2.1-mile trail and some optional rock scrambling) and the other on Iron Mountain, which you can get to in a steep 1.7 miles or as a 6-mile loop that includes the Cone Peak Trail and a section of the historic Santiam Wagon Road. That last road is of interest in itself; some 20 miles remain of this 19th-Century military road, much of which is being developed for multiple users, including "drivers of vintage vehicles and wagons," according to the Willamette National Forest.

For information on all of these activities and plenty more, stop by the Sweet Home Ranger District (it's right on US 20), visit the forest's website at www .fs.fed.us/r6/willamette, or call them at 541-367-5168.

So the "real" fishing is below the dam, and the "real" hiking is a bit up the road, so what's that little park in between all about? Simple: real nice camping.

MAP

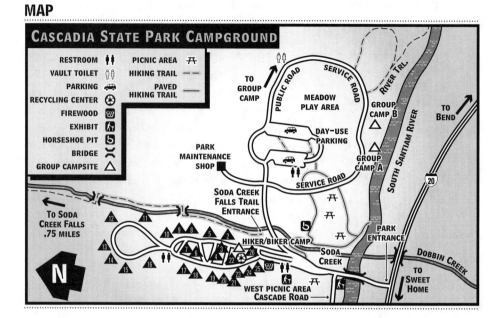

CASCADIA STATE PARK CAMPGROUND

RESTROOM	PICNIC AREA	
VAULT TOILET	HIKING TRAIL	
PARKING	PAVED HIKING TRAIL	
RECYCLING CENTER		
FIREWOOD		
EXHIBIT		
HORSESHOE PIT		
BRIDGE		
GROUP CAMPSITE		

TO GROUP CAMP

PUBLIC ROAD

SERVICE ROAD

RIVER TRL.

MEADOW PLAY AREA

GROUP CAMP B

TO BEND

DAY-USE PARKING

PARK MAINTENANCE SHOP

SOUTH SANTIAM RIVER

GROUP CAMP A

SODA CREEK FALLS TRAIL ENTRANCE

SERVICE ROAD

20

To SODA CREEK FALLS .75 MILES

HIKER/BIKER CAMP

PARK ENTRANCE

SODA CREEK

DOBBIN CREEK

TO SWEET HOME

WEST PICNIC AREA
CASCADE ROAD →

GETTING THERE

Cascadia State Park is
14 miles east of
Sweet Home on US 20.

GPS COORDINATES

UTM Zone (WGS84)	10T
Easting	0541324
Northing	4916134
Latitude	N 44.39731°
Longitude	W 122.481099°

02
FRISSELL CROSSING CAMPGROUND

> *The drive getting to Frissell is as much a part of the adventure as the camping experience itself.*

WHEN YOU DRIVE ALONG THE Aufderheide Memorial Drive (named for a former Willamette National Forest supervisor) on your way to Frissell Crossing, try not to think about what I did: lions and tigers and bears . . . and flying monkeys, and wicked witches. Oh, my!

I happened to be alone. I didn't stop with *The Wizard of Oz,* either. I was Little Red Riding Hood eluding the Big Bad Wolf; I was Gretel without Hansel; I was Scout from *To Kill A Mockingbird* coming home from the Halloween party in her ham costume.

It's easy to let your imagination run wild as you wind along the Aufderheide, whether you approach it from the South Fork McKenzie River side on the north at Blue River or from the North Fork Middle Fork Willamette on the south at Westfir. Some of you will read that sentence at least twice, puzzling over the route. The road, 65 miles long, follows in modern style the pioneering wagon route established by miners and loggers in the late 1800s. As it rises and falls through dense old-growth forest and passes over a low-elevation saddle between the two river drainages, a rich mosaic of historical, geological, and cultural significance is revealed. It would be easy to fill a week absorbing it all between backcountry exploration and roadside edification.

If you don't have that kind of time but still want to get the most out of what the Aufderheide has to offer, take the auto tape tour. The Forest Service provides free-of-charge either a cassette or CD that you can pick up and drop off at various locations on both the north and south entry points to the drive. To my mind, this is a far better idea than having your nose buried in a guidebook (excluding this volume, of course). For one thing, it's kind of dangerous to read and drive at the same time. Second, you can't always prepare in advance

RATINGS

Beauty: ☆ ☆ ☆ ☆ ☆
Privacy: ☆ ☆ ☆
Spaciousness: ☆ ☆ ☆ ☆ ☆
Quiet: ☆ ☆ ☆ ☆ ☆
Security: ☆ ☆
Cleanliness: ☆ ☆ ☆
Insect control: ☆ ☆

if your camping tendencies are as spontaneous as mine. So, read my book first, refer to it when you've stopped at a viewpoint, but keep the tape running while you're driving. I hope this tape tour signals a trend for other agencies, which may elect to manage their scenic byways in a similar fashion. I've always thought similar narration would be a great addition to train travel, too, but that's a different conversation.

Frissell Crossing Campground sits at about the one-third mark on the Aufderheide—from its northern terminus—along the South Fork McKenzie River, which has made a quick descent from its source in the Mink Lake Basin. Although you'll pass several other campgrounds along the route, Frissell Crossing has one thing most others don't: piped water. The camping sites are situated well away from the main road, too, which I always prefer.

Minimally developed sites are spread around an open meadow, retaining in ambience the true essence of the Aufderheide and the primarily roadless wilderness land surrounding the campground. A high canopy of old growth Douglas fir further lends to the sense of space at Frissell Crossing, while generous low-growing vegetation creates a gentle buffer between campsites and adds just the right measure of privacy without claustrophobia. The McKenzie passes through grassy, rhododendron-shrouded banks on the campground's southern border.

With only 12 sites, it's unlikely you'll ever feel crowded, but sites 6 and 7 on the eastern edge of the campground loop are the most removed from the main activity area. During the week, it's not unlikely that you would have the place to yourself. When I visited in mid-August, only three spaces were taken. Certainly no guarantee, but the Aufderheide, one of the first 50 drives in the country to receive federal scenic byway designation in 1988, is not among the more heavily traveled routes in Oregon.

Use Frissell Crossing as a base camp for hiking forays into a multitude of wilderness areas. Due east is the south-central sector of the Three Sisters Wilderness, which laps over into the western Cascades and is far less traveled than its northern counterpart. This region

KEY INFORMATION

ADDRESS:	Frissell Crossing Campground c/o McKenzie River Ranger District 57600 McKenzie Highway McKenzie Bridge, OR 97413
OPERATED BY:	Hoodoo Recreation Services for Willamette National Forest
INFORMATION:	(541) 822-3799 or (541) 822-3381 (ranger district)
OPEN:	May–September
SITES:	12
EACH SITE:	Picnic table, fire grill
ASSIGNMENT:	First come, first served; no reservations
REGISTRATION:	Self-registration on site
FACILITIES:	Vault toilets, hand-pumped water
PARKING:	At campsites
FEE:	$12 per night; $6 per additional vehicle
ELEVATION:	2,600 feet
RESTRICTIONS:	*Pets:* On leash only *Fires:* In fire pits only *Alcohol:* Permitted *Vehicles:* RVs up to 36 feet (turn-around space is limited); no hookups *Other:* 14-day stay limit

MAP

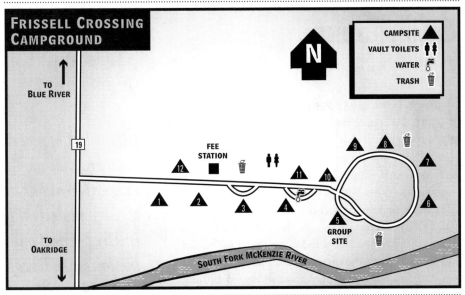

FRISSELL CROSSING CAMPGROUND

TO BLUE RIVER

19

FEE STATION

TO OAKRIDGE

GROUP SITE

SOUTH FORK McKENZIE RIVER

CAMPSITE
VAULT TOILETS
WATER
TRASH

GETTING THERE

From Blue River, take OR 126 4 miles east to FS 19 (Aufderheide Memorial Drive). Turn right, and follow the Aufderheide for 21.5 miles to Frissell Crossing Campground. The campground entrance is on the left. From Westfir, drive north on FS 19 for about 43 miles to the campground on the right.

GPS COORDINATES

UTM Zone (WGS84)   10T
Easting   0567298
Northing   4869083
Latitude   N 43.9718°
Longitude   W 122.161°

of the wilderness is home to a stunning cluster of alpine lakes and the headwaters of the South Fork McKenzie. On Frissell's north side is the French Pete Creek area, the inclusion of which into Three Sisters Wilderness in 1978 preserved some of the most accessible examples of ancient low-elevation old growth. A short drive south of Frissell is the trailhead for access into the northern portion of the Waldo Lake Wilderness.

Driving the Aufderheide requires that you check the gas gauge first. There are absolutely no services along the route, and side trips can eat up your fuel supply. Bring plenty of food rations, too. You just never know where the Willamette's version of the Yellow Brick Road may lead.

Ruby hiking boots, anyone?

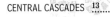

DON'T THINK MOST PEOPLE REALLY GET WALDO LAKE. Ask your friends and neighbors about it, and you'll probably hear something like, "I hear that's nice. I've been meaning to get up there." Well, how does this sound? It's Oregon's second-biggest natural lake (after only Crater Lake) with a surface area of 9.8 square miles. It is also the second deepest lake in Oregon, averaging 128 feet with a maximum depth of 420 feet. It is reputed to be one of the purest lakes on Earth, and when the weather is calm you can see 120 feet down into it. It is also ringed by old-growth forest and wilderness, with mountain views, trails all over the place, no motor boats allowed, and several great campsites.

The three campgrounds (Islet, North Waldo, and Shadow Bay) are pretty much the same, but since Islet is the smallest we're recommending it. However, they all have the same facilities, basic layouts, and they're all on the shore of the lake, so in the grand scheme of things, it doesn't matter where you camp, just as long as you're at Waldo Lake.

And here's why: The lake itself offers wondrous paddling and sailing opportunities, including to some 50 primitive campsites around the lake. You can also paddle out to Rhododendron Island, which as the name suggests is covered with rhodies. They bloom in early summer—unfortunately, so do the mosquitoes—and the island is about 1.5 miles northeast of the ramp in Shadow Bay Campground. Camping is not allowed on the island.

And then there's the hiking, starting with the Jim Weaver National Recreation Trail, known until 2008 as the Waldo Lake Trail. It follows the shoreline for 22 miles, in the process passing through all the campgrounds and connecting with about a dozen other trails. Some of these, west of the lake, lead into the Waldo

> *Islet is one of several campgrounds on magical Waldo Lake, the second deepest lake in Oregon and one of the purest bodies of water on Earth.*

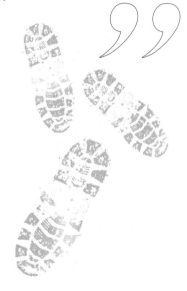

RATINGS

Beauty: ✿ ✿ ✿ ✿ ✿
Privacy: ✿ ✿ ✿
Spaciousness: ✿ ✿ ✿
Quiet: ✿ ✿ ✿
Security: ✿ ✿ ✿ ✿
Cleanliness: ✿ ✿ ✿ ✿ ✿
Insect Control: ✿ ✿ ✿

ADDRESS: c/o Middle Fork Ranger District 46375 OR 58 Westfir, OR 97492

OPERATED BY: Hoodoo Recreation Services for Willamette National Forest

INFORMATION: (541) 782-2283

OPEN: July–September, depending on snow

SITES: 55

EACH SITE: Picnic tables, fire rings

ASSIGNMENT: First come, first served

REGISTRATION: With host

FACILITIES: Compost and vault toilets, piped drinking water, garbage containers, boat launch, recycle center, interpretive sign

PARKING: At sites and in day-use area

FEE: $14; plus $7 per extra vehicle

ELEVATION: 5,400 feet

RESTRICTIONS: *Pets:* On leash only
Fires: In fire pits only
Alcohol: Permitted
Vehicles: RVs and trailers up to 30 feet

Lake Wilderness, with 84 miles of trails and 37,162 lake-filled acres. North of the lake is another trail area with more than a half-dozen other trails, many leading north towards the Taylor Burn Trail Area and, eventually, the southern part of the Three Sisters Wilderness. Passing through all of this, just east of Waldo Lake, is the Pacific Crest National Scenic Trail, which crosses the Willamette National Forest for 118 miles. A favorite spot of mine on that trail is Charlton Lake, which is just off a road east of Waldo Lake. Other worthy goals include Twins Peak (3.3 miles), Maiden Peak (104 miles) and Waldo Mountain Lookout at 6,357 feet. You can hike there and back in a day from North Waldo Campground, but the Forest Service is particularly insistent that you get good maps and know what you're up to. They say the trip "requires several judgment turns and some rather extreme changes in direction. It can be very confusing."

The only other confusing thing around here is why there are still campers in Oregon who haven't been to Waldo Lake.

MAP

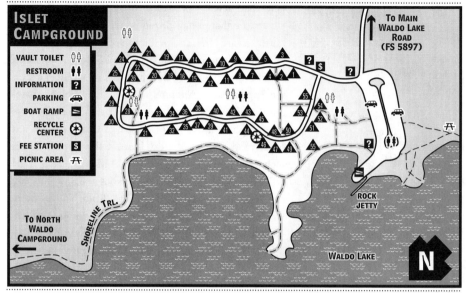

GETTING THERE

From Oakridge, go east on OR 58 for 25 miles to the Waldo Lake Road (FS Road 5897). Follow Waldo Lake Road for 11 miles to FS Road 5898. Continue on FS Road 5898 to Islet Campground.

GPS COORDINATES

UTM Zone (WGS84)	10T
Easting	0579949
Northing	4844363
Latitude	N 43.748°
Longitude	W 122.007°

> *Deep blue waters, azure skies, brilliant green marshes and a snow-capped volcano comprise the scene at Mallard Marsh—one of the prettiest campground settings in this book.*

FOR REASONS UNKNOWN but perfectly accept-able to me, Mallard Marsh gets short shrift in much of the literature about the Central Oregon Cascade Lakes region. Perhaps because the campground name doesn't reflect its location on Hosmer Lake? Perhaps because the term marsh implies a soggy, bug-infested ordeal? Perhaps because Western-ers just can't accept the idea of Atlantic salmon being introduced into their pristine waters? Or maybe just because there are so many camping options in this Mecca for outdoor adventure?

Whatever the reason, I am going to raise aware-ness by saying that Mallard Marsh is likely one of the prettiest campground settings you'll find listed in this book. It has lots of competition from countless other lakes in the region, too, but for one reason or another, none measure up to the outstanding tent camping fea-tures of Mallard Marsh. I know that's saying a lot, but it's hard to deny the exquisite combination of Hosmer Lake's deepest blue waters, azure skies, brilliant green marsh grasses, and colorful waterfowl, topped off with a snowstreaked volcano cone as the backdrop. It sim-ply doesn't get much more picturesque!

The campground itself maintains a very natural countenance to further add to its charm. Driving in past the busy boat launch, you can pick your spot as you pass between the sites, roughly half on the lakeside and the others discreetly tucked on little knolls and in slight depressions. All of the sites are situated under tall stands of lodgepole pine, Douglas fir, and mountain hemlock, with heavy undergrowth of salal, laurel, and huckle-berry providing effective natural screening for privacy. The sites along the lake tend to be a bit more open and enjoy the morning sun's rays earlier. The sites set back receive filtered sunlight all day long and probably are less mosquito-prone.

RATINGS

Beauty: ☆ ☆ ☆ ☆ ☆
Privacy: ☆ ☆ ☆ ☆ ☆
Spaciousness: ☆ ☆ ☆ ☆ ☆
Quiet: ☆ ☆ ☆ ☆ ☆
Security: ☆ ☆ ☆ ☆
Cleanliness: ☆ ☆ ☆ ☆ ☆
Insect control: ☆ ☆

In general, the spaciousness of the sites and the generous greenbelts between them lend a delightfully uncrowded feel to the camping experience at Mallard Marsh, even at the height of a busy summer week. When I pulled into a lakeside drive-through site and walked down to check out the general lay of the land, I could barely see my car not more than 10 yards away!

In this setting, Hosmer Lake is a sport fisherman's dream, but it's one that comes with a few regulations. In order to challenge the wily Atlantic salmon and brown trout that ply the lake's waters, only fly-fishing with barbless hooks is allowed. Nonmotorized boats are the approved mode of travel.

While sailboaters and windsurfers head for Elk Lake when the wind is up, Hosmer is ideal for muscle-powered water travel (i.e. kayaks and canoes) that better suit the quiet ambience of the place anyway. Encompassing only 160 acres, Hosmer makes it easy to spend a lazy afternoon exploring the bordering wetlands and taking in a little birdwatching. Don't forget the binoculars.

The Cascade Lakes region is home to many high-country rambles if the trail calls you out of your lakeside comfort. From the Cascade Lakes Highway, you can satisfy your explorer's urge with trailheads in all directions. Quite possibly, you'll be following along routes established by the early trappers and adventurers who left their indelible historical mark on the region. You could easily spend a full week just on the trails of the Three Sisters Wilderness (due west of Hosmer Lake), discovering one alpine lake gem after another and getting your boots dusty on a section of the Pacific Crest Trail in one of its easiest wilderness access points. From some of the higher vantage points, you can practically watch the weather patterns changing overhead as this is a meeting point for air currents where rapid climatic transition occurs.

Like many of the ancient landmarks that give Oregon its remarkable diversity, the Cascade Lakes region was defined geologically by cataclysmic events that occurred millions of years ago. Unlike many other parts of Oregon, the contours of the landscape, the composition of the soils, and the nature of the vegetation make it possible to view many of Central Oregon's

KEY INFORMATION

ADDRESS:	Mallard Marsh Campground c/o Bend/Fort Rock Ranger District 1230 NE Third Street, Suite A-262 Bend, OR 97701
OPERATED BY:	High Lakes Contractors for Deschutes National Forest
INFORMATION:	(541) 383-4000
OPEN:	May–late September
SITES:	15
EACH SITE:	Picnic table, fire pit
ASSIGNMENT:	First come, first served; no reservations
REGISTRATION:	Self-registration on site
FACILITIES:	Vault toilets, no piped water, boat launch nearby
PARKING:	At campsites
FEE:	$6
ELEVATION:	5,000 feet
RESTRICTIONS:	*Pets:* On leash only *Fires:* In fire pits only *Alcohol:* Permitted *Vehicles:* 22-feet RV size limit, no hookups *Other:* Electric boat motors only

MAP

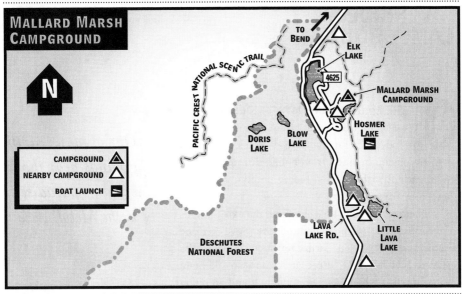

MALLARD MARSH CAMPGROUND

TO BEND

ELK LAKE

4625

MALLARD MARSH CAMPGROUND

PACIFIC CREST NATIONAL SCENIC TRAIL

DORIS LAKE

BLOW LAKE

HOSMER LAKE

N

CAMPGROUND

NEARBY CAMPGROUND

BOAT LAUNCH

LAVA LAKE RD.

LITTLE LAVA LAKE

DESCHUTES NATIONAL FOREST

GETTING THERE

From Bend, follow signs for the Cascade Lakes Highway (FS 46) west around the north side of Mount Bachelor for 35.5 miles. At FS 4625, turn left and drive 1.3 miles to the campground, which will be on your left. You'll bypass Elk Lake on your way to Mallard Marsh. If heading north on the Cascade Lakes Highway, take FS 4625 to the right about 4 miles beyond the Lava Lake Road. At the Y, turn right down the gravel road; turn left just before the boat launch area and you're there.

treasures up close. A good place to start is the Lava Lands Visitor Center or High Desert Museum in Bend. Spend an afternoon there and you'll leave much better prepared for understanding the wonders that await.

One word of warning if you intend to do some daytripping. The closest services to Mallard Marsh are either in Bend or LaPine, and it is easy to lose track of time and distance out here. Make sure you've got a full gas tank.

GPS COORDINATES

UTM Zone (WGS84)   10T
Easting   0597631
Northing   4868605
Latitude   N 43.9641°
Longitude   W 121.783°

05
RIVERSIDE
CAMPGROUND

OH, THE MAGICAL AND MYSTERIOUS Metolius. It wells up clear and bright from an underground spring at the base of Black Butte and provides one of the finest trout habitats around (catch-and-release fly-fishing only) before emptying into the Deschutes River.

There are varying theories about the exact origins of this headwater phenomenon, but the prevailing one seems to be that ancient earth movements blocked the original Metolius and forced it to find an alternate route. It took a while, but it eventually found an outlet at the base of Black Butte. Today, it bubbles and burbles at a rate of 50,000 gallons per minute (right before your very eyes!) to create one of the coldest and clearest rivers in Oregon.

That's why trout like it so much. However, there was a time when salmon sought its cooling waters, too. The word Metolius derives from mytolyas, a term that showed up in a nineteenth-century Pacific Railroad survey report. The reference is to a variety of salmon that is no longer found in the river. Fishermen, on the other hand, will be in plentiful supply if you come to the Metolius at the height of the fly-fishing season. The number of campgrounds on or near the Metolius is staggering, and they are there primarily to serve the abundance of anglers. In addition to Riverside, campers can choose from Camp Sherman, Allingham, Smiling River, Pine Rest, Gorge, Allen Springs, Pioneer Ford, and Lower Bridge.

Riverside is notable in that it has only walk-in sites, which are spacious, grassy, and well-situated under stands of majestic old ponderosa pine. Parking spaces are numbered to correspond with campsites, each within a reasonable distance of the other, but the best sites (those closest to the river) will suddenly seem a long way away if you've got a lot of heavy, cumbersome gear. A small wheelbarrow would be quite useful.

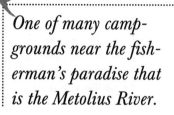

One of many campgrounds near the fisherman's paradise that is the Metolius River.

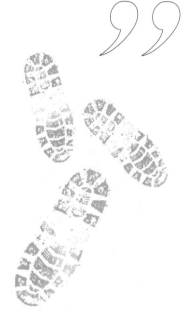

RATINGS

Beauty: ✿ ✿ ✿ ✿
Privacy: ✿ ✿ ✿
Spaciousness: ✿ ✿ ✿ ✿
Quiet: ✿ ✿ ✿ ✿
Security: ✿ ✿ ✿
Cleanliness: ✿ ✿ ✿
Insect control: ✿ ✿ ✿ ✿

KEY INFORMATION

ADDRESS: Riverside Campground c/o Sisters Ranger District P.O. Box 249 Sisters, OR 97759

OPERATED BY: Hoodoo Recreation Services for Deschutes National Forest

INFORMATION: (541) 549-7700

OPEN: May–September

SITES: 16

EACH SITE: Picnic table, fire grill; some shade trees

ASSIGNMENT: First come, first served; no reservation

REGISTRATION: Self-registration on site

FACILITIES: Vault toilets, hand-pumped water

PARKING: At access road, roughly 200–400 yards from campground

FEE: $10; $5 per additional vehicle

ELEVATION: 3,000 feet

RESTRICTIONS: *Pets:* On leash only *Fires:* In fire pits only *Alcohol:* Permitted *Vehicles:* 21-foot RV size limit, no hookups *Other:* 14-day stay limit

This area of central Oregon is characterized by warm—even hot—and dry summers and cold, snowy winters. Upland areas have been known to receive as much as 20 feet of snow, and many trails will be blocked well into May. The terrain is laid with a volcanic base, out of which spills a dazzling collage of crystalline streams, creeks, and rivers. Ancient lava flows, dormant and deteriorated craters, sparkling inlays of obsidian, rugged basalt cliffs, flat-topped mesas and buttes, and numerous lakes dot the landscape.

Dominating the landscape in various stages of geologic splendor are the snowcapped peaks to the west. In order from north to south, they are: Mount Jefferson, Mount Washington, North Sister, Middle Sister, South Sister, and last but not least, despite its forlorn name, Broken Top.

Hiking is one of the best ways to fully appreciate the diversity of this region. There are actually four distinct geographic zones all observable at once: the high-alpine slopes of the volcanoes, with meadows of wildflowers and crumbling lava rock; subalpine forests of ponderosa pine and mountain hemlock nourished by cascading streams and glacial lakes; steep-walled canyons that protect the last of the old-growth fir; and arid pockets of lodgepole pine interspersed with bear grass.

Besides foot travel, other ways to take in the scenery are on horseback and mountain bike. Retrace the routes of such early-day explorers as Lewis and Clark, Kit Carson, and John Fremont on the Metolius-Windigo Trail. Outfitters in Sisters can help you with any hoofed mode of travel.

For cyclists, a 30-mile loop trip along the crest of Green Ridge provides panoramic views of the Cascades. It's a climb of 1,700 feet to the top, and it would be advisable to have a map of the route handy as you ride. This is good advice for anyone who plans to explore places not in the immediate vicinity of FS 14 along the Metolius. There is a crazy network of spur roads that can easily lead you astray if you don't know your way around.

I can't in good faith recommend the Metolius as a boating choice, although it is set up delightfully for water-based recreation. Be aware that the opposite side

MAP

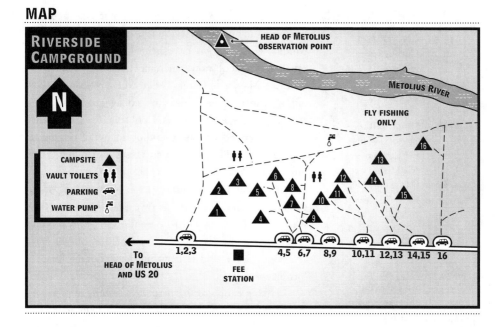

RIVERSIDE CAMPGROUND

N

HEAD OF METOLIUS OBSERVATION POINT

METOLIUS RIVER

FLY FISHING ONLY

CAMPSITE ▲
VAULT TOILETS
PARKING
WATER PUMP

To
HEAD OF METOLIUS
AND US 20

1,2,3

FEE STATION

4,5 6,7   8,9   10,11 12,13 14,15 16

of the Metolius at Riverside is private land and should be respected as such. Farther downstream, the Warm Springs Tribe has jurisdiction over a contentious stretch of the river. If you're looking for a float, I suggest somewhere else or you may be looking at a fight! Check with the Sisters Ranger Station for the latest in this prickly situation and alternate options.

Highlights of a stay at Riverside Campground include short walks to Metolius Spring and Jack Creek Spring, the Metolius River Canyon near Camp Sherman, and the Wizard Falls Fish Hatchery (a surprisingly beautiful setting, unlike most hatcheries).

GETTING THERE

Take SR 126/US 20 (Santiam Highway) north of Sisters to its intersection with FS 14 (Camp Sherman Road). Turn right, and follow FS 14 around the base of Black Butte to FS 900. The camp is less than a mile north on this road. There are some services in Camp Sherman.

GPS COORDINATES

UTM Zone (WGS84)   10T
Easting   609531
Northing   4919921
Latitude   N 44.4243°
Longitude   W 121.624°

06
SCOTT LAKE
CAMPGROUND

> *A little bit of paradise between two wilderness areas, with a lake to swim in and no room for RVs.*

NO MATTER HOW MANY PLACES you camp in Oregon, you're still going to have the experience you may have at Scott Lake. You arrive in a place of such natural beauty, such peace and tranquility, that you can't believe you've never been here before—or that it's so void of people.

I can think of three reasons why so few people camp at Scott Lake, and two of them will work to your advantage. One is that it is almost completely without services: no drinking water, no cut firewood, no parking at the sites. Another is that all the sites are walk-in, which means no RVs and no people who think "walk-in" means "backpack." So these are good things, right?

If you want to know the third reason so few people go, visit in July and check out the mosquito population. In all my conversations with Forest Service Rangers, I have never heard such fear and dread in one's voice as when somebody was telling me about the mosquitoes at Scott Lake in July. So put this one down for mid-August, at least—which works, because that's when the flowers in the nearby wilderness areas will be blooming.

That's right: wilderness areas. A rough guess is that Scott Lake Campground is, as the crow flies, one mile from the Mount Washington Wilderness (52,000+ acres, 28 lakes, one volcano at 7,794 feet) and half a mile from the Three Sisters Wilderness (242,000+ acres, 260 miles of trails, countless lakes, three volcanoes over 10,000 feet).

We could fill a book about the beauty of these two areas—in fact, it's been done, several times over. What we want to convey is this: for the person who seeks peace, quiet, and scenery in their tent camping, Scott Lake is the best place to be if you're exploring Mount Washington and Three Sisters. With tent-only sites scattered around the shore of broad, shallow Scott

RATINGS

Beauty: ☆ ☆ ☆ ☆ ☆
Privacy: ☆ ☆ ☆ ☆ ☆
Spaciousness: ☆ ☆ ☆ ☆ ☆
Quiet: ☆ ☆ ☆ ☆ ☆
Security: ☆ ☆ ☆ ☆
Cleanliness: ☆ ☆ ☆
Insect Control: ☆ ☆

Lake, and others in the trees, you are almost guaranteed to have some space all to yourself. Scott Lake is actually shaped kind of like a big number 3, with sites dotting the left side of the lake. So from the parking area at the Benson Trail trailhead, which is as far north as you can drive, you can walk straight towards the visible water to look for sites, or you can follow the wide trail north to others at the mid section of the "3," or you can go even farther along the trail and look for more spots farther up.

The views from the lowest section are the best; you'll be looking right across the lake at the Three Sisters. The lake isn't much for fishing, but, on the other hand, the little fish in there will probably hit anything. So kids might get a kick out of it. For swimming, you'll need to pick your spots to get in, because the shoreline is shallow and mucky in some spots. On the other hand, motorized craft is banned, so if you can haul a canoe, kayak, inner tube, or some other such thing up there, you can get out on the lake and cruise around.

But back to the wilderness areas. You should certainly stop at the big ranger station in McKenzie Bridge on the way up to get maps, but without moving your car, you can start at Scott Lake and go 1.5 flat miles to Hand Lake or take the other, slightly tougher trail to Benson Lake (1.5 miles), the Tenas Lakes (3 miles) or 6,116-foot Scott Mountain (4 miles) for some serious views. Just across OR 242, and down a half mile or so, you'll find the Scott Trailhead and the Obsidian Trailhead; both of these trails lead about five miles up to the Pacific Crest National Scenic Trail in a world of unmatched meadows, creeks, and mountain scenery. Much of it lies within the Obsidian Special Permit Area, which requires a permit to spend the night in. It's free, but you'll need to get one in advance from the McKenzie River Ranger District.

Even without all that, it's hard to imagine a nicer day in Oregon than hiking around in one of these mountainous wilderness areas, then coming back to Scott Lake and your quiet, peaceful, view-packed campsite. Just don't go in July!

KEY INFORMATION

ADDRESS:	c/o McKenzie River Ranger District 57600 McKenzie Highway McKenzie Bridge, OR 97413
OPERATED BY:	Willamette National Forest
INFORMATION:	(541) 822-3381
OPEN:	July–October
SITES:	14 walk-in tent sites
EACH SITE:	Picnic table; fire ring
ASSIGNMENT:	First come, first served
REGISTRATION:	None as of 2008 (see Fee below)
FACILITIES:	Vault toilet, no drinking water
PARKING:	Along the road, up to 200 yards from sites
FEE:	$5; Northwest Forest Pass or other interagency pass would suffice
ELEVATION:	4,800 feet
RESTRICTIONS:	*Pets:* On leash only *Fires:* In fire pits only *Alcohol:* Permitted *Vehicles:* Cars only; sites are walk-in

MAP

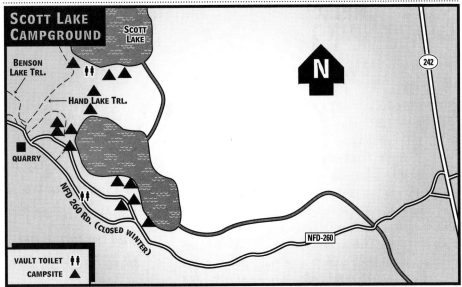

GETTING THERE

From McKenzie Bridge, travel east on OR 126 for 3 miles to OR 242. Follow OR 242 for 14 miles to the campground.

GPS COORDINATES

UTM Zone (WGS84)   10T
Easting   0588756
Northing   4895986
Latitude   N 44.2117°
Longitude   W 121.889°

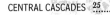

IT'S EASY TO SLIP INTO HYPERBOLE when discussing the North Umpqua River. To many Oregonians, and to fisherman all over the country, just the words "North Umpqua" evoke sighs, bringing to mind crashing, crystalline waters in a forested canyon, with fish, waterfalls, and magical scenery everywhere.

There are, as one might imagine, campsites all along the Rogue-Umpqua National Scenic Byway, also known in these parts as OR 138. Most of these campsites are run by the Forest Service, but Susan Creek is a BLM site, and is probably the most developed BLM site you'll ever visit. It's a long way from rustic, with landscaped sites, showers, an amphitheatre with ranger-led programs, and two hosts for just 29 sites.

Still, it is quite serene, and it is right in the "sweet spot" of the North Umpqua: too far upstream for the inner-tube crowd, too far downstream for most of the whitewater crowd, right on the banks of the North Umpqua, and shaded by massive Douglas firs. And even though a ranger I spoke with told me it's full every weekend and most days, too, he also said it maintains a quiet, "family camping" atmosphere.

A dozen of the sites at Susan Creek are overlooking the emerald green North Umpqua, where fishing is allowed with flies only. Hiking trails leave both ends of the campground, one headed downstream to a free day-use area and 50-foot Susan Creek Falls and the other, which is barrier-free, headed upstream to a "Watchable Wildlife Site" where you can scan the river for eagles, osprey or migrating coho or chinook salmon or sea-run cutthroat trout.

Of course, as nice as the area around Susan Creek is, the larger area around it is truly one of the loveliest corners of Oregon. More than 30 miles of the North Umpqua are designated as Wild and Scenic, and the river alone is a mecca for outdoor fun. Aside from the

Even in a state filled with beauty, few places can touch the North Umpqua River. And no campground there has it all like Susan Creek.

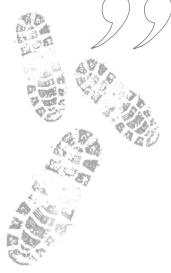

RATINGS

Beauty: ✿ ✿ ✿ ✿ ✿
Privacy: ✿ ✿ ✿
Spaciousness: ✿ ✿ ✿
Quiet: ✿ ✿ ✿
Security: ✿ ✿ ✿ ✿ ✿
Cleanliness: ✿ ✿ ✿ ✿ ✿
Insect Control: ✿ ✿ ✿ ✿

ADDRESS:	c/o BLM Roseburg 777 NW Garden Valley Boulevard Roseburg, OR 97471
OPERATED BY:	Bureau of Land Management
INFORMATION:	(541) 440-4930
OPEN:	Mid-April– mid-November
SITES:	31
EACH SITE:	Picnic table, fire pit, plenty of shade
ASSIGNMENT:	First come, first served
REGISTRATION:	With host
FACILITIES:	Showers, flush toilets, piped water, amphitheatre, river access, two camp hosts
PARKING:	At sites
FEE:	$14; $4 per additional vehicle
ELEVATION:	940 feet
RESTRICTIONS:	*Pets:* On leash only *Fires:* In fire pits only *Alcohol:* Permitted *Vehicles:* RVs and trailers up to 25 feet

fishing, floating the river offers everything from Class I and II (novice) rapids to Class IV (dangerous and requiring scouting). You don't need a permit to float the river, but you do need to know what you're doing, especially above Susan Creek. No matter your skill level and ambition, start by calling the BLM number listed above or the North Umpqua Ranger Station at (541) 496-3532 for up-to-date conditions. A quick Internet search will turn up several commercial rafting operations for the bigger-adventure stuff.

And that's just the river! The hiking in this area is also outstanding, highlighted by the 79-mile North Umpqua Trail which follows the river from Rock Creek (about 10 miles below Susan Creek) to its source at Maidu Lake, high in the Cascades in the shadow of Mount Thielson, and just a mile from the Pacific Crest National Scenic Trail. The trail is divided into 11 segments, broken up by access points which, in some cases, are also campgrounds or recreation sites on their own. There is an excellent brochure available from the Forest Service (the North Umpqua District Office is in Glide).

One of the great features of the trail is that it's across the river from OR 138; this means that from Susan Creek Campground, the closest access to the trail is about 10 miles downstream at Swiftwater Park or five miles upstream at Wright Creek Trailhead. It's above Toketee Lake that the trail leaves the highway for good, following the river through a section called the Dread and Terror Segment—named by some folks that got lost up there decades ago. By all accounts, it's the most beautiful part of the trail and also passes by Umpqua Hot Springs.

As if all this weren't enough, there are shorter trails all over, leading to various meadows, waterfalls, and volcanic features. And OR 138 leads 51 miles up to Diamond Lake (see Thielsen View Campground, page 142 for details) and then another 50 miles to Crater Lake National Park (see Lost Creek Campground, page 130).

So when you're camping at Susan Creek, you're literally surrounded by beauty and adventure. On the other hand, when you're camping at Susan Creek, you might just decide to stay right where you are.

MAP

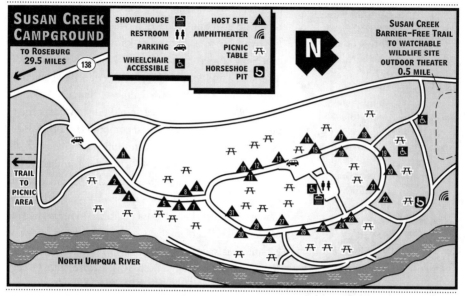

SUSAN CREEK CAMPGROUND

TO ROSEBURG
29.5 MILES 138

SHOWERHOUSE		HOST SITE	H
RESTROOM		AMPHITHEATER	
PARKING		PICNIC TABLE	开
WHEELCHAIR ACCESSIBLE		HORSESHOE PIT	

N

SUSAN CREEK
BARRIER-FREE TRAIL
TO WATCHABLE
WILDLIFE SITE
OUTDOOR THEATER
0.5 MILE

TRAIL
TO
PICNIC
AREA

NORTH UMPQUA RIVER

GETTING THERE

From Roseburg, follow
OR 138 east for 29 miles
to the campground.

GPS COORDINATES

UTM Zone (WGS84)	10T
Easting	0491808
Northing	4794568
Latitude	N 43.3039°
Longitude	W 123.101°

08
THREE CREEK AND DRIFTWOOD CAMPGROUNDS

> *The last 2 miles will challenge your driving skills—and patience— but your reward is a high-altitude tent camper's paradise.*

IF ONE COULD CHOOSE A CAMPSITE via aerial surveillance and parachute in, Three Creek and Driftwood would top my list. I would set my sights on site 17 at Driftwood and "Geronimoooo!" Beam me up in a week, Scotty . . .

Three Creek Lake is a spectacularly beautiful, high-altitude gem that offers a quality tent-camping experience. It's so great, in fact, that I'm giving you a choice of two campgrounds. Driftwood is the nearer to Three Sisters by about a mile (making it a winner in my mind), and Three Creek is at the road's end. Driftwood sprawls around the north shore of Three Creek Lake with 17 sites (12 for tents only). and Three Creek is tucked in on the south side with a cozy 10 sites. Both campgrounds charge the same fee ($12), both are at the same elevation (6,600 feet), and both are quite rustic (without piped water but with garbage service).

Driftwood is accessed off the main road, FS 16, by a short spur to the right. Go for one of the campsites around the farthest perimeter of the lake and you will be ensconced in what feels like your own private reserve, with lots of vegetation and tree cover all around. The drill for these sites is to park your car up above and pack your gear down to the tent site, situated well back from the lake's edge. In fact, most of the sites have their parking space well away from the actual tent-pitching and campfire area. I like this design as it maintains the immediate surroundings outside your tent in a very natural state.

Sites along the spur road closer to the main road are more open, trading heavy vegetation for more of a beachy feel. I saw fishermen on the shore in front of their campsite relaxing in camp chairs with fishing lines extended out into the lake. Maybe not the most die-hard anglers, but they were getting their money's worth out of the campsite!

RATINGS

Beauty: ✩ ✩ ✩ ✩ ✩
Privacy (Three Creek): ✩ ✩ ✩
Privacy (Driftwood): ✩ ✩ ✩ ✩
Spaciousness: ✩ ✩ ✩ ✩
Quiet: ✩ ✩ ✩ ✩ ✩
Security: ✩ ✩ ✩ ✩
Cleanliness: ✩ ✩ ✩ ✩ ✩
Insect Control: ✩ ✩ ✩

At Three Creek Campground, the sites are arranged on either side of the small loop road. Privacy is not as characteristic here, although all sites share a general feeling of being off the beaten path (well-beaten, as a matter of fact). There are a few sites closer to the lake that have the appearance of constant RV wear and tear. Avoid these and choose one of the sites perched on the hillside overlooking the lake.

Most people come to Three Creek Lake for the fishing. But with the massive presence of Tam McArthur Rim, which blocks the view of the craggy peaks in the Three Sisters Wilderness just beyond, you know you could be on the brink of a classic alpine adventure. Three Sisters Wilderness is one of the most heavily traveled areas of Central Oregon. It's also one of the larger tracts at 285,202 acres, and because access points from the north tend to be limited to a few spur roads off FS 16, this section of Three Sisters can be surprisingly lonely.

The trailhead for Tam McArthur leaves from Three Creek Lake adjacent to Driftwood Campground, and since you can see where you're headed, the only way out is up. Once you've reached the top of the rim, however, the trail flattens out. The best views of the Three Sisters cluster (North, Middle, and South Sister, as well as Broken Top Mountains) are a little farther along the trail. Numerous link trails will take you to an assortment of alpine lakes and more views of the heart of the Cascades.

Except for the last couple miles of FS 16, the drive up to Driftwood and Three Creek is not particularly eventful or memorable. The valley floor falls away quickly, but what views can be had are mostly in the rearview mirror or filtered through the lodgepole and ponderosa pines that line this highway. Sit back, enjoy the open road in front of you, and hold onto your teeth for the last couple of miles (which can get bumpy in late summer). Then, you've arrived, have your fill of lake fishing, mountainous hiking, and breathtaking vistas.

Okay, Scotty, I'm ready!

KEY INFORMATION

ADDRESS:	Three Creeks Lake Campground c/o Sisters Ranger District P.O. Box 249 Sisters, OR 97759
OPERATED BY:	Hoodoo Recreation Service for Deschutes National Forest
INFORMATION:	(541) 549-7700
OPEN:	Late May–mid-October, depending on snow level
SITES:	18 at Driftwood; 11 at Three Creeks Lake
EACH SITE:	Picnic table, fire grill; some shade trees
ASSIGNMENT:	First come, first serve; no reservations
REGISTRATION:	Self-registration on site
FACILITIES:	Vault toilets, no piped water, garbage service
PARKING:	At campsites
FEE:	$12; $6 per additional vehicle
ELEVATION:	6,600 feet
RESTRICTIONS:	*Pets:* On leash only *Fires:* In fire pits only *Alcohol:* Permitted *Vehicles:* 20-foot RV size limit, no hookups *Other:* 14-day stay limit, nonmotorized boats only

MAP

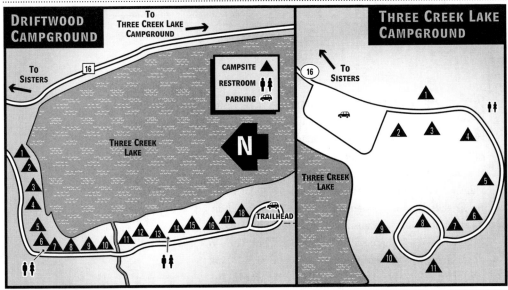

GETTING THERE

From US 20 in Sisters, turn south on FS 16 and drive 17 miles up, up, up to the campground

GPS COORDINATES

UTM Zone (WGS84)   10T
Easting   0610213
Northing   4883979
Latitude   N 44.1007°
Longitude   W 121.623°

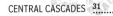

TUMALO STATE PARK CAMPGROUND

FOR ME, THREE DAYS AT TUMALO STATE PARK turned out to be one of the few luxurious extended stays I allowed myself in a madcap summer and fall of feverish campground research. So, if you're in the mood for a little extra campground comfort and want a well-managed compound with excellent facilities, peace of mind when daytripping, and location, location, location, you absolutely cannot beat Tumalo.

For certain, there will be RVs here, but Tumalo does offer a separate tent-camping area (although I think it could use improvement, if that's the right word). The tent camping loop is to the left of the ranger office as you enter the campground driveway. It's a rather small area by comparison to the Loops B and C above, but the tent sites are closest to the Deschutes River, which makes the environment seem more natural. However, the sites themselves are basic, fairly tight together, don't offer a lot of privacy as result of their adjacency, and have awkwardly situated tent pads in many cases.

Up above in the main camp complex, there are two loops, and, if possible, it's best to grab a spot on the outside loop for more privacy. Don't plan on many spaces being available on short notice on summer weekends. If you know the dates you expect to be in the Bend area, it's best to make a reservation. However, there is a new, very specific cancellation policy in the Oregon campground system. Remember to have the cancellation terms clarified when making your reservation.

In fact, it was a lack of a reservation that got me in trouble at Tumalo right off the bat. I arrived with a plan to make Tumalo my base camp for exploring the numerous more rustic tent-camping options in the vicinity—and maybe cram in a golf game at a particular course I had heard good things about. I was hoping to stay five days.

I decided to indulge in the ultimate base camp luxury; I sprang for a yurt for the first time (to report to

> *Go ahead. Indulge yourself. You have my permission, and Tumalo is the place to do it.*

RATINGS

Beauty: ✿ ✿ ✿
Privacy: ✿ ✿
Spaciousness: ✿ ✿ ✿ ✿
Quiet: ✿ ✿
Security: ✿ ✿ ✿ ✿ ✿
Cleanliness: ✿ ✿ ✿ ✿ ✿
Insect control: ✿ ✿ ✿ ✿

KEY INFORMATION

ADDRESS: Tumalo State Park
64120 O.B. Riley
Road
Bend, OR 97701

OPERATED BY: Oregon State Parks

INFORMATION: (541) 388-6055;
www.oregon
stateparks.org

OPEN: Year-round

SITES: 54, plus a hiker/
biker section

EACH SITE: Picnic table, fire
grill; some shade

ASSIGNMENT: First come, first
served or by res-
ervation (recom-
mended in high
season) at (800)
452-5687 or www
.reserveamerica
.com

REGISTRATION: Self-registration

FACILITIES: Flush toilets,
separate solar-
powered shower
building, play-
ground, firewood
and ice for sale; 23
full-hookup sites,
7 yurts, 2 group
tent areas, hiker/
biker camp

PARKING: At campsites

FEE: May–September,
tent sites $17,
hiker/biker $4;
October–April,
tent sites $13,
hiker/biker free.
$5 per additional
vehicles

RESTRICTIONS: *Pets:* On leash only
Fires: In fire grills
Alcohol: Permitted
at campsites only
Vehicles: 30-foot RV
size limit
Other: 14-day stay
limit

my readers, of course). Somehow, I managed to find yurt availability for three consecutive nights—surely the work of the camping gods, because on the fourth day, they conferred again and agreed, "Don't be greedy. You're outta here!" My yurt days may have been short-lived, but my regard for the structures is long-term. They are deserving of every accolade they receive, and may be the affordable answer when good tent camping goes bad.

Fortunately, I was able to complete my research in time and determined that Tumalo was, indeed, an ideal base camp for dandy expeditions in all directions. A morning hike up above Tumalo Falls, an afternoon mountain-bike ride along the Metolius River, an evening gawk at the sunset from Smith Rock, a nighttime frolic in a Bend pub (I said this was my indulgent stint).

Aside from a surplus of RVs (which is every developed campground's plight in my estimation) and an uninspiring tent camping loop, the only notable drawback to Tumalo is the road noise from US 20. It carries over the treetops and above the Deschutes canyon, settling on the campground. Long-haul trucks ferrying goods east and west across the Cascades travel SR 20 with great regularity—and at all hours of the day and night. On a stiller than still night, the truck sounds are a reminder that Tumalo is not necessarily tent camping at its finest, but maybe at its most convenient. And sometimes, that's just what you need.

MAP

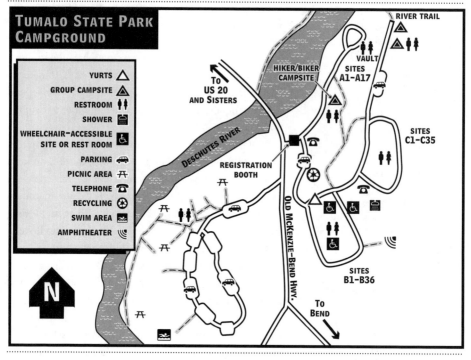

TUMALO STATE PARK CAMPGROUND

YURTS	△
GROUP CAMPSITE	△
RESTROOM	♦♦
SHOWER	🚿
WHEELCHAIR-ACCESSIBLE SITE OR REST ROOM	♿
PARKING	🚗
PICNIC AREA	⛱
TELEPHONE	☎
RECYCLING	♻
SWIM AREA	🏊
AMPHITHEATER	(((

RIVER TRAIL

To US 20 AND SISTERS

HIKER/BIKER CAMPSITE

VAULT SITES A1–A17

DESCHUTES RIVER

REGISTRATION BOOTH

OLD McKENZIE–BEND HWY.

SITES C1–C35

SITES B1–B36

To BEND

N

GETTING THERE

From Bend, take US 20 west towards Sisters. Turn left on Old Redmond-Bend Highway. Turn right on O.B. Riley Road (also known as Old McKenzie–Bend Highway), and wind your way through a few sharp corners and sudden drops. At night, this little stretch of road is surprisingly dark. The campground entrance is on the right just before crossing the bridge over the Deschutes River. Total driving distance from intersection of US 97 and SR 20 in Bend is roughly 5 miles.

GPS COORDINATES

UTM Zone (WGS84)	10T
Easting	0633521
Northing	4887544
Latitude	N 44.1289°
Longitude	W 121.331°

10
WILDCAT CAMPGROUND

A small and lightly traveled territory, Mill Creek Wilderness is right outside your tent's back flap with a variety of hiking options— minus the crowds.

A PLEASANT DRIVE WINDS THROUGH a scenic little valley dotted with neat ranch houses and summer cabins. A lazy stream wanders along, with lush meadow grasses softening its banks. Cattle graze, birds flit, the road rises gently but steadily around each tree-lined bend, and . . . Whoa, Nellie! What the heck is that?!

The sight of lonely Steins Pillar rising 350 feet above the treetops across the valley is not quite what you'd expect in an otherwise pastoral scene, but there it is. A rather prominent vestige of ancient volcanic activity exposed after millions of years of wear and tear, Steins Pillar seems almost comically out of place. Unlike its counterparts, Twin Pillars and Whistler Peak, it was the unwitting victim of bad location when the Mill Creek Wilderness was formed by the 1984 Oregon Wilderness Act. All those years standing out there by itself and it turns out to be only 3 miles shy of where they drew the boundary line! It's unfortunate that there wasn't a way to include Steins Pillar within the protected area. I'll have to ask a ranger for the story, or maybe you can find out for me.

You can view Steins Pillar from a wayside pullover on Mill Creek Road, but there's a fair amount of private land between you and the spire. It takes the right kind of lens to capture the enormity of the pillar on film from this vantage point. If you want to take the detour to view Steins Pillar up close before continuing on up to Wildcat, look for the Steins Pillar sign about a mile past where Mill Creek Road turns to gravel. Turn right, and follow this road sharply up for a little more than 2 miles. The hike in is about 2 miles as well and of average difficulty. Bring a water bottle.

Meanwhile, back at Wildcat . . . The campground is another 5 miles up Mill Creek Road and sits at the intersection of Mill Creek proper and its East Fork. The

RATINGS

Beauty: ✿ ✿ ✿
Privacy: ✿ ✿ ✿ ✿
Spaciousness: ✿ ✿ ✿ ✿
Quiet: ✿ ✿ ✿ ✿ ✿
Security: ✿ ✿ ✿
Cleanliness: ✿ ✿ ✿
Insect control: ✿ ✿ ✿

southwest boundary of the Mill Creek Wilderness is veritably at your tent's back flap. There are few other campgrounds in this book that afford such close proximity to wilderness or so promotes a sense of quietude. Campsites are arranged in a loop with a blend of high desert grasses, aspen, and pines against a backdrop of sun-browned canyon slopes. With the East Fork of Mill Creek babbling through, it's quite a pretty yet primitive setting. The locals will tell you this is one of the best places to cool off from the searing desert heat down below. Having driven in across east central Oregon's John Day River basin, I can wholeheartedly testify to that claim.

The higher you go, the cooler it will get. And the fewer people you'll find. The Mill Creek Wilderness is miniscule by comparison to most of Oregon's other wild lands, but it is the largest of three in the Ochoco Range (Bridge Creek and Black Canyon are the others). Despite this and its modest notoriety for quizzical rock formations, the Mill Creek Widerness often gets overlooked by residents of the Bend/Redmond/Prineville metropolis, who typically migrate west into the Cascades or even further east into the heart of the Blue Mountains. The rock-climbing crowd has turned its fascination northwest to Smith Rock outside Terrebonne, and that reduces the public pressure on Mill Creek's attractions as well.

Given the small stature of the wilderness, its 21 miles of trails can be traversed in no time. On the other hand, once you're here, you might consider taking the opportunity to dawdle since you're not required to canvass the land in record time. You'll get reasonable exercise, though, with three main trails in the system linking to each other in a range of elevations from 3,700 feet (at the campground) to as high as 6,200 feet.

And although it's cooler than the stifling desert, it's still plenty hot and dry, so carry a lot of water.

A word of warning about the East Fork of Mill Creek and its tributaries while on the subject of water: Don't drink from the stream. It may look innocent enough—and how easy it would be to scoop up a palmful while you're heading up the trail to Twin Pillars. But keep in mind that free-ranging cattle are allowed

KEY INFORMATION

ADDRESS:	Wildcat Campground c/o Lookout Mountain Ranger District 3160 NE 3rd Street Prineville, OR 97754
OPERATED BY:	Ochoco National Forest
INFORMATION:	(541) 416-6500
OPEN:	Mid-April– late October
SITES:	17
EACH SITE:	Picnic table, fire grill; some shade trees
ASSIGNMENT:	First come, first served; no reservations
REGISTRATION:	Self-registration on site
FACILITIES:	Vault toilets, piped water
PARKING:	At access road, 200–400 yards from campground
FEE:	$8; $3 per additional vehicle
ELEVATION:	3,700 feet
RESTRICTIONS:	*Pets:* On leash only *Fires:* In fire pits only *Alcohol:* Permitted *Vehicles:* 30-foot RV size limit, no hookups *Other:* 14-day stay limit

MAP

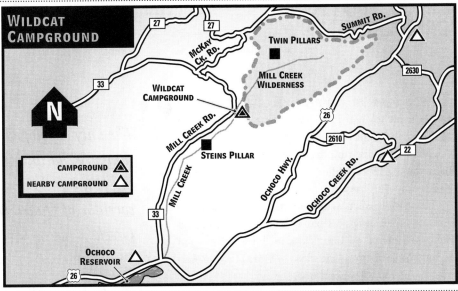

GETTING THERE

From Prineville, head east on US 26 for 9 miles to Mill Creek Road (FS 33). Turn left, and follow the road for approximately 10 miles to the campground.

GPS COORDINATES

UTM Zone (WGS84)   10T
Easting   692741
Northing   4923620
Latitude   N 44.4402°
Longitude   W 120.578°

inside the boundaries of Mill Creek and they have proven to be a nuisance to the natural environment, including the water.

Hopefully, you'll see more wildlife than cattle in your rambles through Mill Creek Wilderness. It's likely that you will, as the level of human traffic is not heavy enough to make native creatures unduly wary. You'd probably rather not run into a black bear or mountain lion (although both live here), but you may be lucky enough to glimpse elk, mule deer, and a variety of birds—the pileated woodpecker thrives on fallen old-growth ponderosas here and wild turkeys roam the lower elevations.

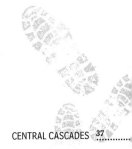

11
YELLOWBOTTOM CAMPGROUND

IF YOU PLAN TO CAMP AT YELLOWBOTTOM and you want to take the scenic route first, come in from the US 22 connector on FS 11. This brings you along the ridge-running, breathtaking Quartzville Backcountry Byway, allegedly one of the least traveled byways in Oregon.

I certainly can't argue with that. When I made the crossing in late August, I passed a handful of cars and only encountered anything close to "busy" when I got beyond Yellowbottom and close to Green Peter Reservoir on the route's western end.

If for no other reason than simply as a tribute to the collection of public and private interests working cooperatively to manage this region, the Quartzville Creek Corridor passes with flying colors. What other 50-mile stretch qualifies as dam-controlled, wild and scenic, historic, and recreational under the auspices of five different agencies? This alone is a modern miracle.

Yellowbottom Campground sits nearly equidistant from both ends of the Quartzville Byway and is the only developed campground within the Wild and Scenic portion of Quartzville Creek, falling under the Bureau of Land Management jurisdiction. Wedged into the right angle formed by Yellowbottom Creek falling from the north and Quartzville Creek running in an east-west parallel with the road, the campground has 20 sites laid out in an intelligent use of the natural geography. It is hard to find a site that seems inappropriate or awkwardly placed. The entire compound evokes simultaneously backcountry wildness and sense of order that is classic BLM—something to do with that "less is more" approach to recreational resources.

Even so, this is one of the more developed BLM campgrounds I came across in my research travels. One would have to refer to Yellowbottom as practically upscale in comparison to most, and this is where the

> *The only developed campground within the Wild and Scenic corridor of Quartzville Creek.*

AU: check this: A proposal was in the works to raise the site fee to $12 for the 2009 season. 503-315-5991

RATINGS

Beauty: ✪ ✪ ✪ ✪ ✪
Privacy: ✪ ✪ ✪
Spaciousness: ✪ ✪ ✪ ✪ ✪
Quiet: ✪ ✪ ✪ ✪ ✪
Security: ✪ ✪ ✪ ✪ ✪
Cleanliness: ✪ ✪ ✪ ✪ ✪
Insect control: ✪ ✪ ✪

ADDRESS: Yellowbottom
Campground
c/o BLM Salem
District Office
1717 Fabry Road SE
Salem, OR 97306

OPERATED BY: Bureau of Land
Management

INFORMATION: (503) 375-5646

OPEN: Memorial Day to
Labor Day

SITES: 22

EACH SITE: Picnic table, fire
grill; shade trees

ASSIGNMENT: First-come,
first-served; no
reservations

REGISTRATION: Self-registration
on site

FACILITIES: Vault toilets,
piped water,
garbage service,
firewood for pur-
chase, camp host,
small hiking trail,
swimming

PARKING: At campsites;
maximum 2 per
site with overflow
parking available

FEE: $8; $5 per addi-
tional vehicle.

ELEVATION: 1,500 feet

RESTRICTIONS: *Pets:* On leash only
Fires: In fire pits
only
Alcohol: Permitted
Vehicles: No
restrictions,
however smaller
trailers and RVs
recommended
Other: 14-day stay
limit; no gathered
wood more than
1 inch in diame-
ter; entrance gate
locked 10 p.m. to
7 a.m.

sense of order is evident. There is a woodshed for firewood, a pump house for water, a power building—for powering what I don't know, and even a small cabin from which the camp host (who is usually on site for the month of August only) distributes literature. Across the Quartzville Road from the overnight camping is the day-use/picnic area, which can be a bit of a hubbub on a sultry summer afternoon. Word has spread of the spectacular swimming hole on the Quartzville here. Bodies sprawl on every available sun-warmed rock surface after a quick plunge in becomes an even quicker scramble out. Quartzville Creek is clear, clear, clear but cold, cold, cold.

For a campground that sports an odd level of organization, the basic amenities (two sets of vault toilets) are not exactly situated in the best proximity to most of the campsites (it can be a long walk in the middle of the night, in other words). The same goes for the piped water. While the best sites for privacy are those backed up against the north slope of the campground (4, 5, 6, 8, 9, and 11), they are the ones where you'll want to consider filling up one container and emptying another (if you know what I mean) before the campfire dies out.

Old growth fir, western red cedar, and rhododendron are the most noticeable permanent residents around Yellowbottom. The Rhododendron Trail, which loops around the north side of the campground boundary, is evidence of their peaceful coexistence and can be observed with a short but robust hike. Longer hikes are not far away in the petite and little-traveled Middle Santiam Wilderness. Here is believed to be the largest remaining stand of old-growth forest in the western Cascades. Consider that piece of information for a minute or two. If you don't make it there on this trip, make sure you put that on your list of things to do sometime next year. The trailhead into the northern sector of the Middle Santiam is accessed off of FS 1142, a right-hand turn not more than 2 miles east of Yellowbottom.

The Quartzville Corridor is truly a gold mine (literally and figuratively), laden with opportunity whether your visit is an afternoon drive, a day picking huckleberries, an overnight gathering around a campfire, a week lost among old-growth giants, or a lifetime of

MAP

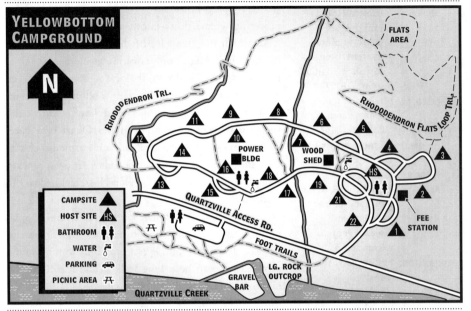

YELLOWBOTTOM CAMPGROUND

N

RHODODENDRON TRL.

RHODODENDRON FLATS LOOP TRL.

FLATS AREA

POWER BLDG

WOOD SHED

HS

HS

CAMPSITE ▲
HOST SITE HS
BATHROOM
WATER
PARKING
PICNIC AREA

QUARTZVILLE ACCESS RD.

FOOT TRAILS

FEE STATION

LG. ROCK OUTCROP

GRAVEL BAR

QUARTZVILLE CREEK

trips, each with something different to offer. Gold mining put this area on the map once and still lures today's amateur fortune-hunters. Primarily, however, it has become the domain of fishermen, boaters, hikers, and berrypickers. For the future, let's hope the legacies we have kept alive and the ones we have created inspire those that follow us.

GETTING THERE

From Sweet Home on US 20 east of Corvallis, turn left (north) on the Quartzville Road (FS 11) and follow it for 24 miles to the campground, which will be on your left. A day-use area and Quartzville Creek are on your right. You can also follow the Quartzville Road west from its eastern connection with OR 22.

GPS COORDINATES

UTM Zone (WGS84)	10T
Easting	0548816
Northing	4937579
Latitude	N 44.5899°
Longitude	W 122.385°

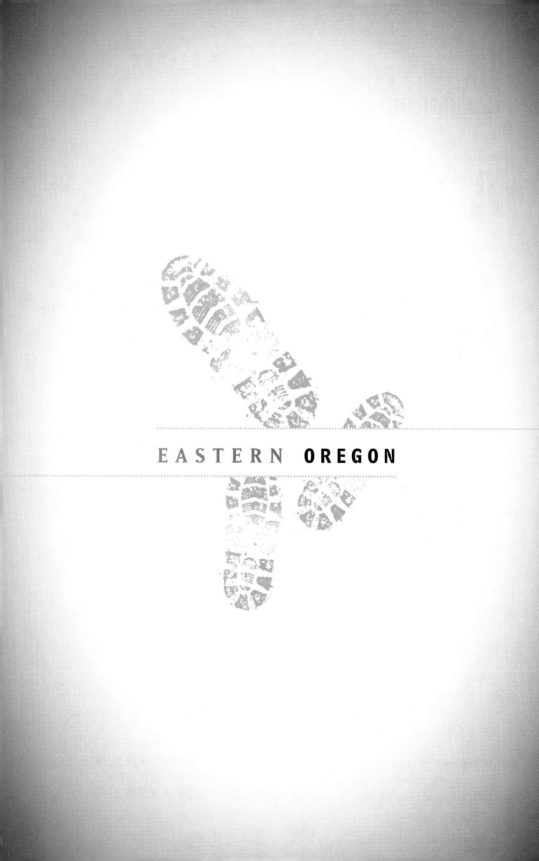

EASTERN OREGON

12
ANTHONY LAKES CAMPGROUND

ANTHONY LAKES CAMPGROUND, at 7,100-foot elevation and only 30 miles northwest of Baker City, is part of the Anthony Lakes Recreation Area, which also includes the much smaller and less developed Mud Lake Campground (with only six sites) and the Anthony Lakes Day-Use Area, popular with valley dwellers seeking a high-altitude escape from the heat far below.

The view from just about any campsite at Anthony Lakes is simply picture-perfect, with the shimmering blue of Anthony Lake contrasting against the dark, sub-alpine forest greens and the rocky, rugged flanks of surrounding Elkhorn Mountains. At this altitude, the fragrances of high-mountain eastern Oregon are irresistible, with pungent notes of woods, earth, and water mingling in the rarefied air. Find one of the sunwarmed, smooth rocks edging the lake, maybe an overhanging tree for a little shade, then dangle a toe or two in the cool waters and indulge yourself.

Unfortunately, if it's a normal summer, the mosquitoes may have you on the go in no time. It's the curse of such a beautiful setting with such a short summer season. They weren't particularly bad in the summer of 2003, but then it wasn't a normal summer, as the snow melt was long gone by mid-July. Winter recreationists are in luck, since they can enjoy the same views mosquito-free at the Anthony Lakes Ski Area right next door and also some of the best powder in Oregon at the highest ski base in the state. Food for thought if you're so inclined and getting eaten alive.

Campsites come in a variety of options if you arrive early. Despite its out-of-the-way feel, this spot does get busy on summer weekends. The main camping area, configured in two loops, sits above and away from the lake as you drive in off FS 73 (Elkhorn Scenic Drive). These are sites 1–27, and I have to say they would not be my first choice. Very tightly spaced, these

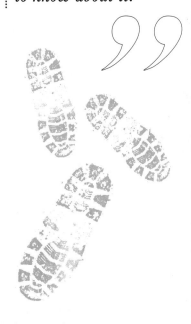

If there's a higher campground in Oregon that has a paved road right to its front door, I'd love to know about it!

RATINGS

Beauty: ☆ ☆ ☆
Privacy: ☆ ☆ ☆ ☆
Spaciousness: ☆ ☆ ☆ ☆
Quiet: ☆ ☆ ☆ ☆
Security: ☆ ☆ ☆ ☆ ☆
Cleanliness: ☆ ☆ ☆ ☆
Insect control: ☆ ☆

KEY INFORMATION

ADDRESS: Anthony Lakes Campground c/o Baker Ranger District 3165 10th Street Baker City, OR 97814

OPERATED BY: Aud and Di Campground Services for Wallowa-Whitman National Forest

INFORMATION: (541) 523-4476

OPEN: April–October, depending on snow levels

SITES: 37; 5 designated for tents, the rest for tents or trailers

EACH SITE: Picnic table, fire grill; some shade trees

ASSIGNMENT: First come, first served; no reservations

REGISTRATION: Self-registration on site

FACILITIES: Vault toilets, drinking water, boat launch, group shelter, group camp sites, picnic areas, reserveable guard station

PARKING: At campsites or in parking lot for walk-in sites

FEE: $8 for tent-only sites; $12 for tent/trailer sites

ELEVATION: 7,100 feet

RESTRICTIONS: *Pets:* On leash only *Fires:* In fire pits *Alcohol:* Permitted *Vehicles:* 14-foot RV size limit *Other:* 14-day stay limit

sites have decent vegetation groundcover, but privacy is at a premium. Try for one that sits on the outside of the loop for the least-crowded feel.

I found the best sites to be the walk-ins (28–32), which are in optimum proximity to lake views, generously spaced, and close enough to parking for easy unloading of gear and provisions. They are, however, staggered on either side of the footpath that circumnavigates the lake, which may get busy when other campers are out for a shoreside stroll.

A string of campsites, numbered 33–39, lies on the far south side of the lake beyond the boat launch. These sites are spaced similarly to the walk-in sites, but being on the flats and closer to the lake may enhance the mosquito presence. They are also closer to the boat put-in, which could mean early morning noise.

Nearby are the original Civilian Conservation Corps campsites, preserved from 1933 when workers were busy getting the ski area ready for opening. It was one of the first in the country and at the time totally modern thanks to the newest invention of the day: the rope tow.

Activities abound in the Anthony Lakes area year-round. South and west of the campground is the Baldy Unit of the North Fork John Day Wilderness, a small, rugged area with hiking options in uncrowded terrain. Access to the Elkhorn Range contained within parts of the wilderness is available via the Elkhorn National Scenic Trail, which departs very near Anthony Lakes. Peaks and buttes in the Elkhorns rise as high as 9,100 feet, offering magnificent vistas of this compact but diverse pocket of the Blue Mountains.

You're likely to see as much wildlife as people; the region supports herds of elk and various deer species, black bear, mountain lions, mountain goats, hawks, and the occasional (seasonal) bald eagle. Consequently, however, it's a popular hunting area in the fall. The North Fork John Day River, designated wild and scenic in one stretch west of Anthony Lakes, is known for its abundant fish populations, including chinook and steelhead migrating in astounding numbers up from the Columbia. Brook trout, Dolly Vardens, and rainbows also thrive in the North Fork.

MAP

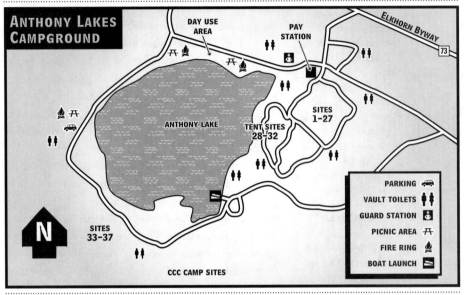

ANTHONY LAKES CAMPGROUND

DAY USE AREA

PAY STATION

ELKHORN BYWAY

73

ANTHONY LAKE

TENT SITES 28-32

SITES 1-27

SITES 33-37

CCC CAMP SITES

N

PARKING	🚐
VAULT TOILETS	👫
GUARD STATION	🚻
PICNIC AREA	🏕
FIRE RING	🔥
BOAT LAUNCH	⛵

Historically speaking, more people frequented this area on a regular basis around the turn of the century than do today. The discovery of gold in the late 1860s combined with a flourishing lumber industry, pioneer ranching, and completion of the transcontinental railroad contributed to a healthy stretch of boom years for towns such as Granite, Sumpter, Austin, and Bourne. Though much has been destroyed by time, fire, and neglect, there are a few buildings scattered throughout the region still standing as tribute to that rough-and-tumble period in Oregon history.

One of the best ways to gain a richer appreciation of the area is to drive the entire Elkhorn National Scenic loop—a 106-mile paved route with marked points of interest along the way. It's a good day-tripping option if you make Anthony Lakes Campground your base.

GETTING THERE

Anthony Lakes is 30 miles northwest of Baker City following US 30 to CR 1146 to FS 73. Follow signs directing you to Anthony Lakes Ski Area or along the Elkhorn Scenic Byway when in doubt.

GPS COORDINATES

UTM Zone (WGS84)   11T
Easting   0402681
Northing   4979681
Latitude   N 44.9639°
Longitude   W 118.234°

> *When one ranger tells you about a secret place, you figure it's worth a look. When two rangers tell you about the spot, you know you've got a keeper.*

BUCKHORN IS A LONG WAY FROM ANYWHERE, not unlike many of the lonely, sacred spots around the Blue Mountains, the Wallowa Valley, and Hells Canyon National Recreation Area. If you're looking for a place to lose yourself, you've found it.

The campground itself is not the centerpiece of the Buckhorn experience; it is simply the place to pitch your tent, come back to in the evening, tell stories over the crackling campfire, and rub your sore feet after a day of hot, dusty trailblazing to which you've willingly subjected yourself. Okay, so you're not exactly the first person who's been out here (or there wouldn't even be this primitive campground), but at Buckhorn you get the feeling that you could be the last person to visit for a long time.

The sense of loneliness begins on the drive up from Enterprise, when you start out on the Crow Creek Road off of OR 82. At indistinctly marked junctions, the road becomes Zumwalt-Imnaha Road, then Zumwalt-Buckhorn Road, then FS 46. There's no one on the road to ask for directions; ranch houses are tucked deep in the folding fields and usually have gated entrances.

All of these anxieties aside, the Zumwalt ranks as a modern-day magic carpet ride. Miles and miles of burnished gold and brown grasslands roll out before you as you climb gently but steadily on a gravel expressway through this magnificent benchland, the smooth contours and rich colors contrasting sharply with the stark, contorted shadowy jumble of the canyons to the east and the jagged, snowcapped peaks of the Wallowas in the rear-view mirror.

The few campsites (five total) that comprise Buckhorn are heavily vegetated (which is a pleasant surprise given the otherwise sparsely shrubbed ground). This is due, in large part, to the presence of Buckhorn Spring,

RATINGS

Beauty: ✿ ✿ ✿
Privacy: ✿ ✿ ✿ ✿ ✿
Spaciousness: ✿ ✿ ✿ ✿
Quiet: ✿ ✿ ✿ ✿ ✿
Security: ✿
Cleanliness: ✿ ✿
Insect control: ✿ ✿ ✿ ✿

a stalwart little underground spurt that creates an oasis of plantlife in this harsh environment. When you drop down to the campground on FS 783 from the main access road (FS 780), which continues on to the lookout, you will feel as though you've stumbled onto a private thicket that could easily be an afternoon resting ground for local deer.

Quickly assessing that primitive is a generous word for Buckhorn Campground, you will also recognize that the beauty of this campground lies in its remoteness, its raw simplicity, and its location a mere hundred yards from the mesmerizing view. The familiar "less-is-more" attitude is a good one to adopt when taking in the wonders from this perch on Oregon's northeastern rim.

By the time you reach the campground, you'll be quite aware that you're near the Buckhorn Overlook. It's less than a mile from the campground, and from there, you actually get two views for the price of one, as the viewpoint sits high above the lower Imnaha River near where it empties into the mighty Snake. Flashes of brilliant sunlight on the river far below catch your eye. Raptors soar in the thermal currents high above. At eye level as far as you can see, ridges and tables and knobs and shelves of varying geophysical proportions and timelines thrust and jut and hunker and lean in an incomparable tableau. It's panorama-plus through a viewfinder, and in all honesty, I've never seen a photograph that did it justice.

It's easy to see why Chief Joseph and his peaceful band of Nez Perce so loved this land—and why the U.S. government wanted control of it, too. Exploitation and misunderstandings ensued, and Chief Joseph was forced out. Hike to Spain Saddle for continuously impressive views of the Imnaha and Snake River Canyons and even the Salmon River deeper into Idaho.

Enjoy Buckhorn for what it was then, is today, and mostly, for what it isn't. Take away an appreciation of some of the most wild, untamed areas of Oregon desperately trying to remain that way, and when it comes time to vote to preserve this special place, do the right thing.

KEY INFORMATION

ADDRESS:	Buckhorn Campground c/o Wallowa Valley Ranger District 88401 Oregon Highway 82 Enterprise, OR 97828
OPERATED BY:	Wallowa-Whitman National Forest
INFORMATION:	(541) 426-5546
OPEN:	May–late September
SITES:	5
EACH SITE:	Picnic table, shade trees; four with fire grills
ASSIGNMENT:	First come, first served; no reservations
REGISTRATION:	Not necessary
FACILITIES:	Pit toilet; no piped water
PARKING:	At campsites
FEE:	None
ELEVATION:	5,200 feet
RESTRICTIONS:	*Pets:* On leash only *Fires:* In fire pits only *Alcohol:* Permitted *Vehicles:* Not recommended for RVs

MAP

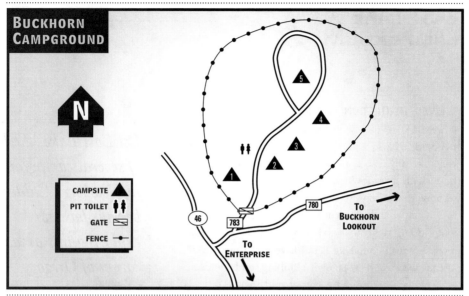

BUCKHORN CAMPGROUND

N

CAMPSITE ▲
PIT TOILET 🚻
GATE ⬛
FENCE ●—

5
4
3
2
1

46
783
780
To BUCKHORN LOOKOUT

To ENTERPRISE

GETTING THERE

Buckhorn is 43 miles northeast of Enterprise (which is east of LaGrande on OR 82). From OR 82, take the Crow Creek Road to Zumwalt Road. Turn right, and continue to FS 46; then turn right again on FS 780. The roads out here aren't particularly well-marked. I had to stop several times to make sure I was taking the correct fork. A good local road map wouldn't be a bad idea. Nearly the entire drive is on fine gravel, so expect a dust cloud following you like a posse in the summer.

GPS COORDINATES

UTM Zone (WGS84)   11T
Easting   0512444
Northing   5066728
Latitude   N 45.754°
Longitude   W 116.84°

14
EAST LAKE CAMPGROUND

I LIVED IN OREGON for almost 12 years before I went to Newberry Volcanic National Monument. Looking back, with shame, I believe the reasoning went like this: "It's a volcanic monument (been to those) with lava flows (seen 'em), geological features, (whatever) and lakes (check).

If this sounds like you, just stop it. Stop whatever you're doing right now and make plans to visit Newberry. It's really amazing. You drive east from US 97, past meadows and trees, ever climbing, and then suddenly you come around a corner and there's this big lake, with forested mountains on the other side. This is Paulina Lake. You keep going a few more miles, past ever more impressive views, and there's another one! This is East Lake.

Combined, these two lakes cover some 2,300 acres; East Lake averages 65 feet in depth, and Paulina averages 170 with a deepest spot around 250 feet. And both lakes are ringed by trails (13 miles in all) offering access to the shorelines.

In other words, if I could have a conversation with myself in the past, I'd say, "Yeah, it's a volcanic monument with two lakes, but you should see the lakes!"

There are seven campgrounds within the monument, and from what I've seen the best are East Lake, Cinder Hill, Little Crater, and Paulina Lake—in that order. I'm concentrating here on East Lake for several reasons; it's the smallest of the bunch (though still fairly large) and offers the most shade and privacy per site. But since they're all first-come, first-served, and since you are going to the Monument at your first chance, start at East Lake, and if it's full, just find someplace else to stay.

Once you're there, here's something to think about. You're inside the caldera of a volcano, and it's about 4 by 5 miles wide. A caldera is what's left when the summit of a volcano collapses (Crater Lake is an

> *Let East Lake, the best of several campgrounds in Newberry Caldera, be your base for exploring this amazing corner of Oregon.*

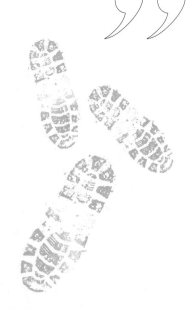

RATINGS

Beauty: ☆ ☆ ☆ ☆ ☆
Privacy: ☆ ☆ ☆
Spaciousness: ☆ ☆ ☆
Quiet: ☆ ☆ ☆
Security: ☆ ☆ ☆ ☆ ☆
Cleanliness: ☆ ☆ ☆ ☆
Insect Control: ☆ ☆ ☆ ☆

KEY INFORMATION

ADDRESS: c/o Bend-Fort Rock Ranger District 1230 NE 3rd Street, Suite A-262 Bend, OR 97701

OPERATED BY: High Lakes Contractors for Deschutes National Forest

INFORMATION: (541) 383-4000

OPEN: May–October

SITES: 29

EACH SITE: Picnic table, fire ring

ASSIGNMENT: First come, first served

REGISTRATION: With host

FACILITIES: Vault and flush toilets, drinking water, boat launch, accessible campsite and toilet

PARKING: At sites

FEE: Regular site $12; lakeside site $14; $6 per additional vehicle

ELEVATION: 6,400 feet

RESTRICTIONS: *Pets:* On leash only *Fires:* In fire pits only *Alcohol:* Permitted *Vehicles:* RVs and trailers up to 26 feet

example), and in this case, the whole Newberry Volcano is about 20 miles wide! The monument is a wonderland of lava flows, cinder cones, hot springs, obsidian flows, lava caves, forests, and trails.

And fish—Really, really big fish. Both Lakes are home to rainbow and brown trout, Atlantic salmon, and kokanee. The biggest brown caught there was 22 pounds, 8 ounces; Paulina Lake holds the state record for a brown at 28 pounds, 5 ounces. Ask at the entrance to the monument for the latest restrictions and regulations.

For hiking, there are more than 60 miles of trails to choose from, ranging from short interpretive trails to the 21-mile Crater Rim Trail, which loops around in the high country, exposing you to wide open views and connections to several other trails, including Paulina Lakeshore (7 miles) and the Paulina Peak Trail.

But why hike to Paulina Peak when you can drive there? The highest point in the monument (7,984 feet) has a 360-degree view that takes in the caldera and both lakes, the south and west flanks of the volcano, the Cascades, the Fort Rock Basin and much of Central Oregon. It's said that on a clear day you can see from Mount Adams in Washington to Mount Shasta in California—a spread of some 350 miles. I haven't driven the 4.1-mile Paulina Peak Road, so I can't attest, but the Forest Service calls it steep, dusty, and "quite rough and precipitous in some places." I also have no doubt that it's worth the trip.

One final note to consider for your rapidly upcoming trip to Newberry Monument: it's bear country, as every page on the Monument website will remind you. Bear visits are said to be fairly common in campgrounds, so do your part by following all the food storage regulations.

And don't let the bear thing—or anything else, for that matter—deter you, because you are going to East Lake, and soon. Right?

MAP

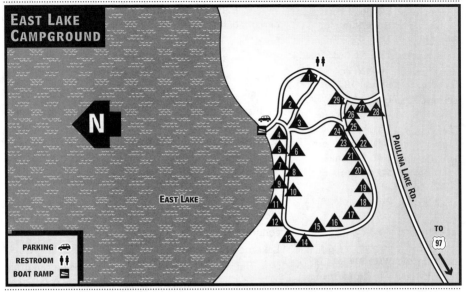

EAST LAKE

PAULINA LAKE RD.

TO 97

PARKING
RESTROOM
BOAT RAMP

GETTING THERE

From Bend, go 23.5 miles
south on US 97, then
16.6 miles east on Rd. 21
(Paulina Lake Road). There
are signs a-plenty.

GPS COORDINATES

UTM Zone (WGS84)   10T
Easting   644191
Northing   4842087
Latitude   N 43.7178°
Longitude   W 121.21°

15
HART MOUNTAIN NATIONAL ANTELOPE REFUGE CAMPGROUND

> *Out where the deer and antelope play, literally, is a little oasis of shade, peace, . . . and hot springs!*

THERE'S OUT THERE, there's really out there, and then there's getting to Hart Mountain Antelope Refuge from the nearest town of Frenchglen, population 11! You follow OR 205 south for about 10 miles, then turn onto a gravel road which the government says "is not maintained for passenger vehicles," and follow it for 37 miles, often washboarded, to the headquarters. Sixty-five miles in the opposite direction is Lakeview; the local metropolis at 2,474 souls.

In between? A whole lot of wide-open beauty. And antelope. And free creekside campsites with hot springs.

Now, the question in your mind might be, "What's this about 'not maintained for passenger vehicles'?" And you're right to ask. But one of your authors applied the 93 Sentra Test—can a 1993 Nissan Sentra handle it?—and the roads from Frenchglen and Lakeview did just fine. And while it's longer, the route from Lakeview is better, so plan on taking that route unless you're already in the Frenchglen/Steens Mountain area (like at Page Springs Campground, page 69).

Now, as for why you should go to Hart Mountain. For starters, have you ever seen antelope? You almost certainly will at Hart Mountain, though it might be from a ways off, so bring binoculars or a telescope. Second, no place in this book—heck, in Oregon—is more wide open and beautiful than Hart Mountain. And yet it's far from being lifeless. Of course, there are the antelope (a.k.a. pronghorn), who are not as shy as you might think; I had to wait for some to walk across Frenchglen Road, and they even posed for photos within 100 feet. If you're really lucky, you'll get to see one run; they can do 45 mph, and their eyes work at the equivalent of 8-power binoculars. The refuge says the eastern area, along Frenchglen Road and Lookout Point is the best place to spot these stars of the refuge.

RATINGS

Beauty: ✿ ✿ ✿ ✿ ✿
Privacy: ✿ ✿ ✿ ✿
Spaciousness: ✿ ✿ ✿ ✿ ✿
Quiet: ✿ ✿ ✿ ✿
Security: ✿ ✿ ✿ ✿ ✿
Cleanliness: ✿ ✿ ✿ ✿
Insect Control: ✿ ✿ ✿

And yet it's not all antelope out there; the refuge hosts 239 species of birds, especially on the western edge at the Warner Wetlands, a series of astonishing lakes at the base of amazing cliffs. (Yes, it's the land of superlatives.) The spring migration season is the highlight here, and the refuge has built several blinds for your convenience. Tougher to spot, but still around, are bighorn sheep, bobcats, and coyotes. And rattlesnakes, so keep an eye and an ear out, and leash that dog!

Among the activities—that is, other than looking around saying "Dang!"—you can hike, ride horses, ride (very sturdy) bikes on the roads, rockhound (for surface rocks less than seven pounds), backpack, and, of course, look for critters.

In the middle of all this dry vastness, Hot Springs Campground is the place to stay. There are two other campgrounds (one for horses) but Hot Springs is where it's at, with 30 sites stretched along two creeks, most of them tucked into little pockets of Aspen trees. It's the very definition of rustic—no water, no fire rings, rough roads, and some sites without tables—but it's also free, and while RVs are allowed, the use of generators is banned. And did we mention the hot springs? There are even three tent-only walk-in sites, but they lack shade and are not in the best part of the campground.

Oh yes, the hot springs! There is one right in the middle of the campground, about five feet deep with room for perhaps six adults at a time. The water is not terribly hot—at least, it wasn't when I visited in October—and in 2008, the refuge actually built a stone wall with some benches around it. Some folks grumbled about this, because part of the charm before was that you were sitting in the springs with a view of everything. But the flip side of that is that everybody had a view of the springs, and as you probably know, most hot springs in Oregon (including this one) are "clothing-optional," and most people opt for no clothing. So I suspect that's why there's now a spiffy, five-foot stone wall around the springs.

After a day spent roaming the high desert, bonding with antelope and migratory birds, and contemplating the vast expanse of blue sky, even a little wall

KEY INFORMATION

ADDRESS:	Hart Mountain National Wildlife Refuge 18 South G Street Lakeview, OR 97630
OPERATED BY:	U.S. Fish and Wildlife Service
INFORMATION:	(541) 947-3315
OPEN:	Year-round, but it might close for snow on occasion, and the refuge's roads could get dicey in winter and spring
SITES:	30
EACH SITE:	Most have a picnic table
ASSIGNMENT:	No reservations
REGISTRATION:	At the entrance
FACILITIES:	A hot spring, pit toilets . . . and not much else
PARKING:	At sites
FEE:	None
ELEVATION:	6,000 feet
RESTRICTIONS:	*Pets:* On leash only *Fires:* Banned during dry seasons, and you'll have to bring your own wood *Alcohol:* Permitted *Vehicles:* RVs and trailers up to 20 feet

MAP

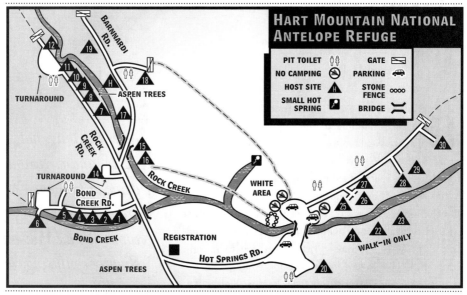

HART MOUNTAIN NATIONAL ANTELOPE REFUGE

PIT TOILET	👫	GATE	⊠
NO CAMPING	🚫	PARKING	🚐
HOST SITE	H	STONE FENCE	○○○○
SMALL HOT SPRING	⚲	BRIDGE	⟩⟨

BARNNARDI RD.

TURNAROUND

ASPEN TREES

ROCK CREEK RD.

TURNAROUND

BOND CREEK RD.

ROCK CREEK

WHITE AREA

BOND CREEK

REGISTRATION

ASPEN TREES

HOT SPRINGS RD.

WALK-IN ONLY

GETTING THERE

From Lakeview, follow OR 140 north, and then east for 32 miles, then turn north onto Plush Cutoff Road. Take this 18 miles to the hamlet of Plush, then pick up Hart Mountain Road for 26 miles to the refuge headquarters. From here, follow signs for 4 miles south to Hot Springs Campground.

around your hot springs shouldn't get between you and a peaceful state of mind.

GPS COORDINATES

UTM Zone (WGS84)   11T
Easting   0278715
Northing   4708674
Latitude   N 42.4988°
Longitude   W 119.693°

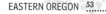

16
HIDDEN CAMPGROUND

A PEACEFUL, BEAUTIFUL, almost poetic setting on the shoulders of the upper Imnaha River, it's even easier to appreciate Hidden Campground after the drive down from Joseph, which I found to be a real test even though it is entirely paved. What starts off as a gentle grade up on Little Sheep Creek Road, with wide views of the Wallowa Valley as it falls away behind you, quickly becomes a twisting, narrow, roller-coaster ride when you turn right onto FS 39 (Wallowa Mountain Loop Road).

Keeping both hands on the wheel is vital as you pass through an area that burned in 1988 and work your way towards the ultimate drop down to the Imnaha River Road, approximately 30 miles from the start of Wallowa Mountain Loop Road. I found the road signs confusing even with a good USGS map. Although the road following the Imnaha both north and south is officially the Imnaha River Road, to the left it is FS 3955 and to the right it continues briefly as FS 39 and then becomes FS 3960. At this intersection, the main road, FS 39, takes an angle left towards its intersection with OR 86. The key is to keep taking rights—never a left—and you will ultimately find your way to Hidden Campground. Perhaps others had similar problems locating the campground and named it accordingly.

The campground itself is not hidden at all. In fact, it is one of the few campgrounds along the Imnaha that offers gorgeous, open sites with lovely tall grasses under towering ponderosa pines and tamarack. Sun filters through the tall trees and a cooling breeze kicks off the fast-falling Imnaha to make for a heavenly combination on a scorching summer day.

Granted, Hidden Campground is about as primitive as they come, with only a picnic table and fire grill at each of its 10 sites. Every site sits well-spaced from its neighbors along the river, so there's no chance of a

> *After the long, hot, dusty, and circuitous drive to Hidden Campground (either way you come, it's all that and slightly confusing, too), you'll just have one thing to say: "Ahhh . . ."*

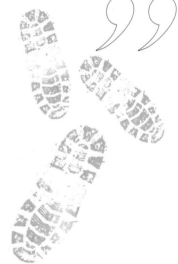

RATINGS

Beauty: ✿ ✿ ✿ ✿ ✿
Privacy: ✿ ✿ ✿ ✿
Spaciousness: ✿ ✿ ✿ ✿ ✿
Quiet: ✿ ✿ ✿ ✿ ✿
Security: ✿ ✿ ✿
Cleanliness: ✿ ✿ ✿ ✿
Insect control: ✿ ✿ ✿ ✿

KEY INFORMATION

ADDRESS: Hidden Campground c/o Wallowa Valley Ranger District 88401 Oregon Highway 82 Enterprise, OR 97828

OPERATED BY: Wallowa-Whitman National Forest

INFORMATION: (541) 426-5546

OPEN: Mid-April– mid-October

SITES: 10

EACH SITE: Picnic table, fire grill; some shade trees

ASSIGNMENT: First come, first served; no reservation

REGISTRATION: Self-registration on site

FACILITIES: Vault toilets, no piped water

PARKING: At campsites

FEE: $5

ELEVATION: 4,400 feet

RESTRICTIONS: *Pets:* On leash only *Fires:* In fire grills only *Alcohol:* Permitted *Vehicles:* Small RVs or trailers OK, no hookups

particularly bad spot despite sparse ground cover. Sites 8, 9, and 10 are located on the loop where outgoing traffic circles by, and may experience a bit more noise as a result. The wind in the trees and the sounds of the river ought to drown out most disturbances, which would be temporary anyway. The Forest Service rates Hidden as a high-use facility, but when I was there in midsummer midweek, there were only two sites taken. Blessedly, there were no RVs, which glutted the more developed campgrounds that I passed on the way in.

Aside from an overkill of four outhouses, there's very little else that interrupts the natural environment. And this is as it should be, since the campground is located within the Hells Canyon National Recreation Area and surrounded by just about every wilderness, wild and scenic, and national forest boundary possible. Immediately west, the officially designated "Wild and Scenic" segment of the Imnaha River plunges out of the Wallowa Mountains. A little further west is the boundary for the Eagle Cap Wilderness and the only trail access into it from this side of the Wallowas (from Indian Crossing Campground at road's end). Due east is Hells Canyon Wilderness and the "Wild and Scenic "Snake River. Beyond that, there's Idaho. This is the southeasternmost boundary of the Wallowa National Forest, and just across the river on the Imnaha's south bank is the northeasternmost corner of the Whitman National Forest.

If you need any guidance on things to do, a hike into the Eagle Cap Wilderness is number one on my list. Next are the Imnaha River Trail and the Imnaha Crossing Trail. Afterwards, make the drive to McGraw Lookout for an unstoppable view over Hells Canyon and some well-placed interpretive plaques and meditation benches. The drive north along the Imnaha River Road leads you to other Hells Canyon overlook points and to the town of Imnaha.

Traveling south along FS 39 and onto OR 86 to the west, the route of the Wallow Mountain Loop Road continues. This is more than a one-day loop from your starting point at Hidden (unless you get a really early start), so you may want to retrace your steps at about Halfway (the name of the town, not the mileage mark) or take OR

MAP

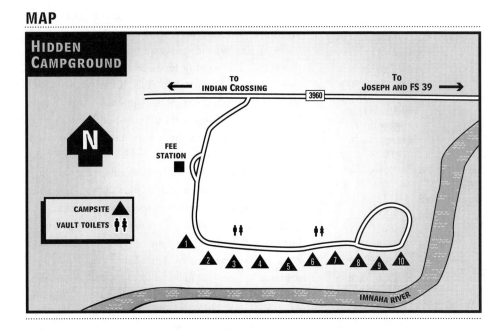

HIDDEN CAMPGROUND

TO INDIAN CROSSING ←

3960

TO JOSEPH AND FS 39 →

N

FEE STATION

CAMPSITE ▲
VAULT TOILETS 👫

1 2 3 4 5 6 7 8 9 10

IMNAHA RIVER

---

86 east to the town of Copperfield for a different perspective of Hells Canyon and a look at Oxbow Dam.

Paddlers are advised that the Imnaha River in the vicinity of Hidden requires expert skills, and even then it may be a foolhardy venture. The river drops very steeply and is log- and debris-choked in many spots, demanding a thorough scouting of the waters before any descents are considered. The buddy system is essential in this technical, remote area.

Another option is fishing; the Imnaha is little-known to most anglers, but it hosts rainbow and bull trout, as well as wild and hatchery steelhead. Trout season is May 27 through October 31; steelhead season on the mainstem Imnaha is in spring, winter, and fall.

GPS COORDINATES

UTM Zone (WGS84)	11T
Easting	0501730
Northing	4995670
Latitude	N 45.1145°
Longitude	W 116.978°

GETTING THERE

From Joseph, take SR 350 (Little Sheep Creek Highway) to FS 39 (Wallowa Mountain Loop). At the intersection with Imnaha River Road (FS 3960), turn right and follow the river to Hidden's entrance on the left. You'll pass several other campgrounds on the Imnaha Road. The driving distance from Joseph is roughly 44 miles; the last 9 are gravel and everything in between is steep, narrow, and twisting. It's very slow going. The lower Imnaha is home to a daunting system of Forest Service roads that all seem to look alike. A good local road map is a must.

17
MARSTER SPRINGS CAMPGROUND

Beneath mountain lakes, above desert and wetlands, under the shade of tall trees by a lovely river

THERE ARE TWO RATHER AMAZING ecosystems in this part of Oregon, and Marster Springs Campground sits right between them. That alone would make it worth visiting, because you can use it as a base for exploring both the desert and wetlands around Summer Lake as well as the high country around Gearhardt Mountain Wilderness and Yamsay Mountain.

But it's also true that Marster, on the banks of the Chewaucan River, is a wonderfully pleasant and quiet campground shaded by tall trees. Even better, most people visiting the area zoom right past it, headed uphill or down on Forest Road 33. Their loss, your gain.

This part of Oregon gets surprisingly little visitation, and, in fact, many of the campgrounds in the area don't see any real crowds until deer hunting season in the fall. This has always seemed odd to me. The area around Summer Lake is home to wide-open vistas, soaring peaks, and even the sprawling wetlands of Summer Lake Wildlife Refuge. The spring-fed Ana River nourishes these marshes, which, in March and April, host vast flocks of ducks, geese, and swans, and, in April and May, see more songbirds and other waterfowl. And, by the way, the typical April day in these parts is mostly sunny with a high around 60. Think about that if you live west of the Cascades!

After birding, stop at Summer Lake Hot Springs, less than an hour from camp; there, you can enjoy 103-degree water in a 15-by-30-foot pool underneath a 1927 bathhouse. (Day use, from 8 a.m. to 9 p.m., is only $5; see **summerlakehotsprings.com** for more information).

Driving uphill from Marster Springs, you're quickly into the high country, and recreation options abound—mostly hiking and scenic driving. The trail cutting through it all—indeed, stretching some 115 miles

RATINGS

Beauty: ✿ ✿ ✿ ✿ ✿
Privacy: ✿ ✿ ✿ ✿
Spaciousness: ✿ ✿ ✿ ✿
Quiet: ✿ ✿ ✿ ✿ ✿
Security: ✿ ✿ ✿ ✿
Cleanliness: ✿ ✿ ✿ ✿
Insect Control: ✿ ✿ ✿

across the Fremont and Winema National Forests—is the Fremont National Recreation Trail. This trail (mostly used by horse riders but also open to hikers) traverses such spectacular lookouts as Winter Ridge (2,000 feet above Summer Lake and 30 miles long!) and 8,196-foot Yamsay Mountain (which offers views from California's Mount Shasta to Oregon's Cascades).

The Fremont Trail also just happens to run right by Marster Springs Campground, across the Chewaucan, which is said to have pretty decent fishing for rainbow and brook trout. The trail can be accessed at Chewaucan Crossing Trailhead, a quarter-mile south on FS 33, where there's an impressive pedestrian bridge.

Many of the trails here, despite their high elevation, tend to melt out by June, meaning you can hike up high here long before you can in the Cascades. But you should also understand that while mosquito season in the Cascades is July, here it's May—and they're incredible, like a living fog. By June they're dying off, the flowers are out in the high meadows, and all is lovely. Grab a map and look for hiking options in Gearhardt Mountain Wilderness (22,000 acres, around 7,500 feet elevation), around Yamsay Mountain, or up on Winter Ridge. Or just drive around, fish, look for beaver ponds and marshes, and enjoy the views.

I should tell you that if you want to camp higher up, there are some nice campgrounds to choose from. Dead Horse Lake and Campbell Lake sit in the hub of a trail network; both were closed in 2008, or they might be described in greater detail here. Smaller and quieter are Lee Thomas and Sandhill Crossing Campgrounds, both on the North Fork of the "Wild and Scenic" Sprague River around 6,300 feet elevation.

I'd recommend either of those if you just want to be up in the mountains in quiet campgrounds. The lakes see more activity, but have more options on site. If you want to be down in the valley, you can pitch your tent at Summer Lake Hot Springs, although there's no shade there at all.

But if you want to be in the middle of it all, in a nice, quiet campground next to a scenic river, head for Marster Springs.

KEY INFORMATION

ADDRESS:	c/o Paisley Ranger District P.O. Box 67 Paisley, OR 97636
OPERATED BY:	Fremont National Forest
INFORMATION:	(541) 943-3114
OPEN:	Open year-round, maintained May 15–October 31
SITES:	10
EACH SITE:	Fire ring, picnic table
ASSIGNMENT:	First come, first served
REGISTRATION:	At entrance
FACILITIES:	Pit toilet, water pump, no garbage service
PARKING:	At sites
FEE:	$6 fee; $2 per additional vehicle
ELEVATION:	4,845 feet
RESTRICTIONS:	*Pets:* On leash only *Fires:* In fire pits only *Alcohol:* Permitted *Vehicles:* RVs and trailers up to 25 feet

MAP

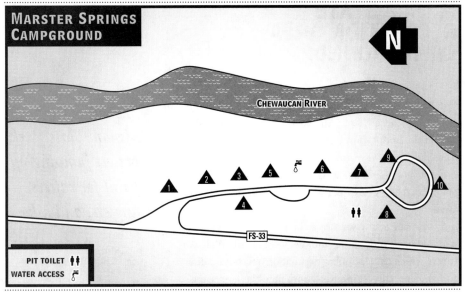

MARSTER SPRINGS CAMPGROUND

CHEWAUCAN RIVER

FS-33

PIT TOILET
WATER ACCESS

GETTING THERE

From OR 31 in Paisley, go south on Mill Street, which becomes Forest Service 33 at a Y junction. Follow FS 33 for 7 miles to the campground on the left.

GPS COORDINATES

UTM Zone (WGS84)   10T
Easting   0696325
Northing   4721718
Latitude   N 42.6229°
Longitude   W 120.606°

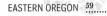

18
MINAM STATE RECREATION AREA CAMPGROUND

IF YOU'RE LOOKING FOR A COZY, SECLUDED campsite, look elsewhere: All of the primitive campsites
in this campground are in a huge open clearing
where you can wave to your neighbors. But don't dis-
count it just yet. What it may lack in privacy, Minam
State Recreation Area certainly makes up for in other
areas.

For starters, it sits pretty in a remote valley on a
steep bank overlooking the whitewater of Wallowa
River, which is a popular destination for both rafters
and anglers. Large pine trees dominate the landscape.

The Indians called this area—which extends from
the mouth of Indian Valley where the Grande Ronde
narrows, down to the confluence of the Grande Ronde
and Wallowa Rivers—"Hunaha." Lochow Lochow,
"lovely little forest," was the central Indian camp for
the Nez Perce, who harvested wild vegetables, fruit,
fish, and game through the summer months.

Two launching points for boaters are located in
the nearby day-use area, and you can even rent a raft at
the nearby store. Some rafters even return from their
runs with tales of bighorn sheep sightings. Anglers will
also enjoy this area, as the river is renowned for steelhead and rainbow trout. You can catch your dinner
and make use of that fire pit back at your campsite.

Water adventures aren't the only thing drawing
visitors; the nearby Wallowa Mountains offer some of
the best all-day hiking and backpacking trails in the state,
making this a perfect spot to set up camp along the way
and return to after a day of hiking. It's also not nearly as
crowded as nearby Wallowa Lake Campground—even
on a holiday weekend you're likely to find an empty
spot. Keep your eyes open, as the area plays host to
wildlife such as bear, elk, and deer. Bear sightings were
a common conversation topic on my visit.

> *Minam State Park is a perfect jumping-off point for rafters, anglers, and hikers.*

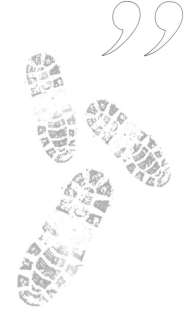

RATINGS

Beauty: ✰ ✰ ✰ ✰
Privacy: ✰ ✰
Spaciousness: ✰ ✰ ✰ ✰
Quiet: ✰ ✰ ✰
Security: ✰ ✰ ✰ ✰
Cleanliness: ✰ ✰ ✰ ✰
Cleanliness: ✰ ✰

KEY INFORMATION

ADDRESS: Minam State Recreation Area 72214 Marina Lane Joseph, OR 97846

OPERATED BY: Oregon State Parks

INFORMATION: (541) 432-8855, (800) 551-6949; www.oregon stateparks.org

OPEN: April–October

SITES: 12

EACH SITE: Picnic table, fire ring

ASSIGNMENT: First-come, first-served; no reservations

REGISTRATION: Self-registration on site

FACILITIES: Vault toilets, piped water

PARKING: At campsites

FEE: $8 May–September, $5 October–April; $5 per additional vehicle

ELEVATION: 2,500 feet

RESTRICTIONS: *Pets:* On leash only
Fires: In fire rings only
Alcohol: Permitted at campsites only
Vehicles: 1 car per site parking
Other: 14-day stay limit

While the campsites may seem a little confusing as you first enter the campground—they aren't well-marked upon first glance and there's no clear-cut difference between one site and its neighbor—there are advantages to this open type of campground. For one thing, it's a prime spot if you're bringing a large group along because your group can camp on the large grassy knolls. Some of the sites offer asphalt tent pads, and most have water nearby. All of the sites offer views of the Wallowa River. A nearby store will stock you up with ice, food, and fishing supplies, but be warned: It tends to close early, so make sure you don't return from an all-day hiking trip with a big thirst, only to be disappointed. It's best to come prepared, but Elgin is only about 10 miles west, so you're not completely out of luck.

If you find yourself recovering from the aches of a long hike or rafting trip, Elgin also offers a unique way to view the valley's majestic scenery—by rail. The Eagle Cap Excursion Train (800-323-7330) offers round-trip rides from nearby Wallowa to Joseph, where you can sit back and enjoy view from the train's Pullman cars. Don't forget to bring your camera.

However you decide to enjoy this natural setting, keep in mind that the climate in Eastern Oregon varies greatly with elevation. The higher up you go, the colder the temperatures and higher the chance of precipitation. If you're visiting the region during the summer months, be prepared for afternoon thunderstorms and chilly evening temperatures. Don't be surprised if you encounter snow on high country trails at any time of year.

MAP

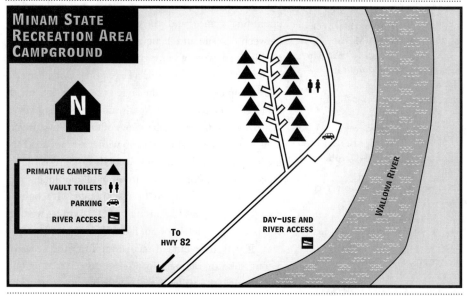

MINAM STATE RECREATION AREA CAMPGROUND

N

PRIMATIVE CAMPSITE ▲
VAULT TOILETS 👤👤
PARKING 🚗
RIVER ACCESS ▤

To
HWY 82

DAY-USE AND
RIVER ACCESS
▤

WALLOWA RIVER

GETTING THERE

From Elgin, drive 13 miles
northeast on US 82, and turn
left (north) at the sign for
Minam State Recreation
Area. Drive 2 miles to the
end of the road and the
campground.

GPS COORDINATES

UTM Zone (WGS84)   11T
Easting   0444457
Northing   5069997
Latitude   N 45.7813°
Longitude   W 117.7145°

19
NORTH FORK MALHEUR CAMPGROUND

> *How does a free campground on the banks of a trout stream in the middle of forest and mountains sound?*

SOMETIMES A CAMPSITE IS JUST THAT: a place where you can camp. That may sound simplistic, but if you were traveling or backpacking, and you were looking for a place to bed down, this is probably what you would want: someplace quiet, out of the way, pretty, in a flat clearing by the side of a lovely river with some fish in it, not many people around, and free.

Well, that's North Fork Malheur Campground: five sites along the banks of a "Wild and Scenic" River, with stuff to do all around you, but also a darn fine place to just, well, camp.

And now, a few words of reverence for the North Fork of the Malheur River. When folks talk about the "health" of a river and an ecosystem, they generally refer to the well-being of some "indicator" species. On the North Fork of the Malheur, which was designated "Wild and Scenic" in 1988, those species are redband trout and, especially, bull trout.

Is a trout just a trout? Well, no. A bull trout, as my fishing friend Craig likes to put it, is a predator. It eats other fish, and as a result, gets really big–up to two feet long and 20 pounds! Craig assures me that hooking one of these "beasts" is the thrill of a fishing lifetime. Now, the bull trout is an endangered species, because it needs a particular habitat to surive: many miles of cold, clear, oxygenated water (which we would call "bubbly") and a situation the Forest Service calls "minimal historic and current activities." That's a government way of saying "nobody messing with it." Well, the North Fork Malheur is serious Bull Trout Country, as many signs around will remind you. It starts its 23-mile course (all protected as "Wild and Scenic") in a glaciated valley filled with ponderosa pines, flowery meadows, and big-time views, then flows among old-growth ponderosa pines through a narrow, rough canyon with walls as

RATINGS

Beauty: ✿ ✿ ✿ ✿ ✿
Privacy: ✿ ✿ ✿
Spaciousness: ✿ ✿ ✿ ✿ ✿
Quiet: ✿ ✿ ✿ ✿
Security: ✿ ✿ ✿ ✿
Cleanliness: ✿ ✿ ✿ ✿
Insect Control: ✿ ✿ ✿ ✿

high as 750 feet. Eventually it joins the Middle Fork Malheur, which is also protected, and together they dance off into the sage and juniper country down below.

And along its scenic way, the North Fork Malheur passes our lovely little campground. And if it's not deer hunting season, you just might have the place to yourself. This is, in part, because the last bit of road is a little rough, but it passed my '93 Sentra Test with flying colors. You'll see some cattle around, too, but they are kept clear of the campground by guards on the road.

A quarter-mile down the road you'll find the trailhead for the North Fork Malheur Trail, which follows the river for 12.4 miles. Fishing is allowed, but bull trout must be released unharmed. Another thing people love to do in this area is ride mountain bikes, as there are old roads all over the place that are no longer suitable for cars. Bikes are also allowed on the North Fork Trail, and motorized vehicles are not. For any of this, of course, you'd want a really good map of the district, so stop in the Prairie City Ranger District office on the way out.

And if you're wondering about the name Malheur, it literally means "bad hour" in French; the name comes from Peter Skene Ogden, who camped on the river with French-Canadian trappers in 1826 and discovered that a cache of furs left there the previous year had been stolen. What he was calling it was the "unfortunate river."

KEY INFORMATION

ADDRESS: c/o Prairie City Ranger District P.O. Box 337 Prairie City, OR 97869

OPERATED BY: Malheur National Forest

INFORMATION: (541) 820-3800

OPEN: May–October, depending on snow

SITES: 5

EACH SITE: Picnic table, fire pit

ASSIGNMENT: First come, first served

REGISTRATION: None

FACILITIES: Pit toilet, no water

PARKING: At sites

FEE: None

ELEVATION: 4,700 feet

RESTRICTIONS: *Pets:* On leash only
Fires: In fire pits only
Alcohol: Permitted
Vehicles: RVs and trailers up to 25 feet

MAP

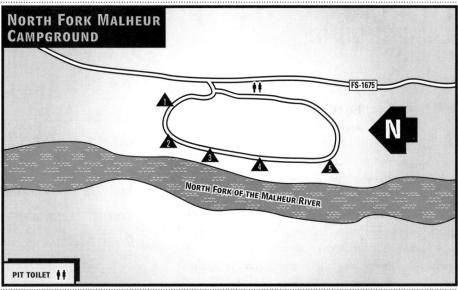

North Fork Malheur Campground

FS-1675

North Fork of the Malheur River

N

PIT TOILET

GETTING THERE

From Prairie City, take County Road 62 (Bridge Street in town) south for 8.5 miles and turn left onto Forest Service Road 13. Follow FS 13 for 16 miles to FS 16 and South Creek Guard Station. Turn right onto FS 16 and go 2 miles to a fork. Here, follow FS 1675 left for 2.4 bumpy miles to the campground.

GPS COORDINATES

UTM Zone (WGS84)   11T
Easting   0389589
Northing   4896015
Latitude   N 44.209°
Longitude   W 118.382°

BEFORE GOING FURTHER, I must first confess that Olive Lake was not initially one of my top 50 campgrounds. Sometimes, the fickle finger of campground-research fate has the last word, and so it was on the day that Olive Lake jumped onto the "A-list."

Fortunately, Olive Lake turned out to be a more than adequate alternative. It has played such an integral role throughout the history of this region, from the early gold-mining days to its contemporary recognition as a valuable focal point for area recreation, habitat restoration, and historical preservation. The combination makes for an interesting blend, offering opportunities to learn and explore in one of the least-traveled areas of eastern Oregon. I apologize for giving it short shrift in the initial overview.

I reached Olive Lake by way of the Elkhorn Scenic Drive out of Baker City, but you can also find it from the north by dropping south on I-395 out of Pendleton or from the west via a more circuitous route off of Highway 26 out of Austin. A good map of the state, county, and Forest Service roads in the lonely outposts of Baker and Grant Counties is a wise traveling accessory if you want to be adventurous with peace of mind.

The campground is shaped like a horseshoe around the north end of the lake, offering either lake-front living or views from just about every site. There are a total of 28 tent sites, 23 of which can also be RV sites. Five sites are walk-in only. There are two group sites and three picnic areas. Sites are gargantuan in size and generously spaced, so have no worries about feeling hemmed in. Low-bush undergrowth is spare, which further enhances the feeling of openness. Lodgepole pines, with their slim trunks, don't clutter the campground yet provide high-canopy relief from the sun on hot days and precipitation on wet ones.

> *Olive Lake benefits from a combination of historical, recreational, and environmental preservation.*

RATINGS

Beauty: ✪ ✪ ✪ ✪
Privacy: ✪ ✪ ✪ ✪
Spaciousness: ✪ ✪ ✪ ✪ ✪
Quiet: ✪ ✪ ✪ ✪ ✪
Security: ✪ ✪ ✪ ✪
Cleanliness: ✪ ✪ ✪ ✪ ✪
Insect control: ✪ ✪ ✪

KEY INFORMATION

ADDRESS: Olive Lake
Campground
c/o North Fork
John Day Ranger
District
P.O. Box 158
Ukiah, OR 97880

OPERATED BY: Umatilla National
Forest

INFORMATION: (541) 427-3231

OPEN: Late May–October

SITES: 28

EACH SITE: Picnic table, fire
grill, shade trees

ASSIGNMENT: First come,
first served; no
reservations

REGISTRATION: Self-registration
on site

FACILITIES: Vault toilets,
no piped water,
2 group sites,
day-use areas

PARKING: At campsites and
at the boat ramp/
dock

FEE: $10 for single sites,
$25 for group sites

ELEVATION: 6,000 feet

RESTRICTIONS: *Pets:* On leash
only, no garbage
service
Fires: In fire rings
only
Alcohol: Permitted
Vehicles: No RV size
limit although not
all sites will
accommodate
large RVs, no
hookups and no
dump
Other: Gas and
electric boat
motors allowed

Many of the campers who occupied sites when I visited had a "settled-in" look about them, suggesting they had been there a long time. Many of these regulars return year after year to their favorite spots and quickly become part of the scenery. According to the camp hosts, the majority of campers who enjoy Olive Lake are repeat customers. Maybe that's why they eyed my car suspiciously when I drove in.

Olive Lake, pitted in its center with an island of trees, sits high in the Greenhorn Range of the Blue Mountains at an elevation of 6,000 feet. The Greenhorn Unit of the North Fork John Day Wilderness can be accessed via a short hike heading southeast from the south end of the lake. The boundary between the Umatilla National Forest and the Malheur National Forest works its way in right angles along high rock buttes and crumbled ridges southwest of the lake. To the north, the largest unit of the North Fork John Day Wilderness encompasses 86,000 acres, creating a protected passageway for the North Fork John Day River and visitors looking to enjoy its "Wild and Scenic" designation.

Recreationally, the lake is a destination for anglers who are allowed to use boats with both electric and gas motors (strange, so close to a wilderness boundary) to chase after their catch. Kokanee, cutthroat, rainbow, and brook trout are the prime fish to catch. A 2.5-mile trail surrounding the lake is an easy evening stroll, but a longer, more challenging hike takes you north and west to Saddle Camp and Ridge. You can hike along the spine of Saddle Ridge or make the crest of Saddle Camp your turnaround point. A loop hike continues down Saddle Ridge and along Lost Creek at various points to return to Olive Lake either via a trail or FS 10. Half of this loop trip winds through designated wilderness where you won't encounter any motorized travel.

Historically, Olive Lake was the water source for the Fremont Powerhouse, which served mining and municipal interests for the first half of the twentieth century. A wood-and-steel pipeline was constructed to funnel water nearly straight down the mountainside to the powerhouse. You can still see parts of the pipeline as you travel along FS 10 or along the aforementioned

MAP

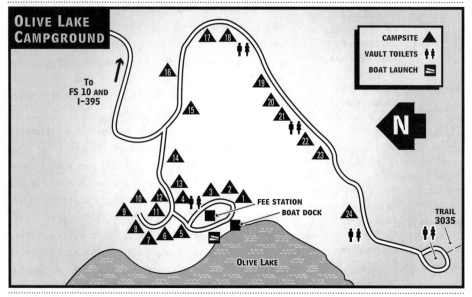

OLIVE LAKE CAMPGROUND

To FS 10 and I-395

- CAMPSITE ▲
- VAULT TOILETS 👥
- BOAT LAUNCH 🛶

N

FEE STATION
BOAT DOCK
TRAIL 3035

OLIVE LAKE

loop hike. The Powerhouse has been placed on the National Register of Historic Places and is open to visitors. The complex includes a caretaker's house and three other cabins. The cabins have been refurbished and are now available to rent.

Olive Lake can be busy in the summer, so it's good to have an alternative close by.

GPS COORDINATES

UTM Zone (WGS84)	11T
Easting	0373984
Northing	4960579
Latitude	N 44.7875°
Longitude	W 118.593°

GETTING THERE

From Pendleton, drive south on I-395 to the turnoff for Highway 244 (51 miles). In the center of Ukiah, turn south on Camas Street (immediately west of the city park). This is part of the Blue Mountain National Scenic Byway. Follow this paved road (it turns into Forest Road 52) for approximately 41 miles to the town of Granite junction. Turn right on FS 10 and in about 3.5 miles this paved road will become gravel. At the Y where that occurs, stay right and head uphill about 8 miles to Olive Lake.

*Of three BLM camp-
grounds in the Steens
Mountain area,
Page Springs is the more
centrally located for day
trips and the only one
open year-round.*

ONE LOOK AT THE SOUTHEASTERN EXPANSE of Oregon, roughly 60 miles south of Burns, and you know you're in a place where country-western music is as common as cornbread. Mile after dusty mile, scraggly sagebrush, twisted juniper, and jagged rimrock share a landscape punctuated only by the hulk of mile-high Steens Mountain. This is the highest fault-block mountain in the nation and a snowcapped beacon for all of southeast Oregon.

The region was once the turf of the largest cattle ranch in the United States. Pete French arrived in the Donner und Blitzen River Valley in 1872 with 120 head of cattle and built an empire that totaled 45,000 cattle and 200,000 acres. Cattle operations still exist in parts of the Steens Mountain area today. But with all the natural wonders to behold, outdoor recreation and tourism are emerging as alternatives to traditional sources of income that are gradually fading away.

Page Springs Campground sits invitingly in the midst of this spectrum. Maintained by the Bureau of Land Management out of its Burns District office, Page Springs is one of three public campgrounds that the Bureau provides for visitors. I prefer it because it is centrally located for interesting day trips, which await in just about every direction. It is also the only one of the three campgrounds that is open all year.

Once you've settled in among the sagebrush and aspens, stretch your legs after the hot, dusty drive and explore the immediate surroundings on a 1.8-mile stroll that follows the meandering Donner und Blitzen River through tall stands of surprisingly lush grasses and other hardy indigenous vegetation. This short path is part of a longer route known as the Desert Trail that will, if the efforts of the national Desert Trail Association are suc-cessful, provide access to some of the most beautiful arid sections of North America between Canada and

RATINGS

Beauty: ✿ ✿ ✿ ✿
Privacy: ✿ ✿ ✿
Spaciousness: ✿ ✿ ✿
Quiet: ✿ ✿ ✿ ✿ ✿
Security: ✿ ✿ ✿ ✿
Cleanliness: ✿ ✿ ✿ ✿ ✿
Insect control: ✿

Mexico. Oregon's contribution to the trail network is 77 miles.

Now that you're warmed up (or cooled down, more accurately), consider the more distant options. If you're visiting the area in summer, you may want to escape the intense, merciless heat with a drive around Steens Mountain National Backcountry Byway. Be sure to fill your gas tank and carry extra water for both you and the car. Humans require a gallon per person per day, I've heard—although that doesn't seem quite adequate around here. Better to carry extra than too little. The road to Steens is quite rough, the entire loop distance is 66 miles, and what minimal emergency services exist are in Frenchglen, which will be well behind you once you set out. The weather can change quickly and dramatically, so be prepared for extremes of wind and precipitation. Snow is not uncommon in midsummer at higher altitudes. One last thing: The road is not recommended for RVs. (Isn't that just a beautiful thing?)

While all this emergency preparedness may sound either overly dramatic or a bit daunting, you'll thank me later. Once you reach the summit of Steens, you'll want to stick around a while and take in all that this magnificently desolate area has to offer. And you'll be making numerous stops along the way, as there are overlooks and short hikes to distract you.

Take your time and enjoy the journey. Think about it: When was the last time you had an opportunity to drive to the top of a 9,773-foot mountain that unabashedly bares so many of its geologic secrets? Witness the effects of glacial activity with such clear-cut examples as Kiger, Little Blitzen, Big Indian, and Wildhorse Gorges—massive U-shaped troughs up to half a mile deep. The mountain is a veritable living laboratory for botanists and biologists, with five distinct habitat zones ringing its slopes.

Wildlife abounds in the Steens Mountain area, and Malheur National Wildlife Refuge just north of Page Springs provides viewing areas from which as many as 280 species of birds and nearly 60 species of mammals have been observed. The refuge's 185,000 acres of lakes, ponds, marshes, and soggy meadows rank it as one of the top havens for breeding waterfowl,

KEY INFORMATION

ADDRESS:	Page Springs Campground c/o Burns District Office 28910 US 20 West Hines, OR 97738
OPERATED BY:	Bureau of Land Management
INFORMATION:	(541) 573-4400
OPEN:	Year-round
SITES:	32
EACH SITE:	Picnic table, fire pit with grill; shade trees
ASSIGNMENT:	First come, first served; no reservations
REGISTRATION:	Self-registration on site
FACILITIES:	Pit toilets, piped water, garbage service, group picnic shelter, limited disabled access
PARKING:	At campsites
FEE:	$8 May–October; $4 November–April
ELEVATION:	4,200 feet
RESTRICTIONS:	*Pets:* On leash only *Fires:* In fire pits only *Alcohol:* Not permitted *Vehicles:* No hookups for RVs or trailers

MAP

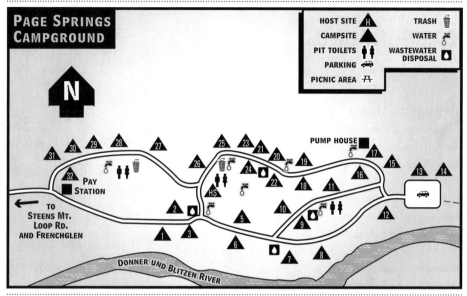

PAGE SPRINGS CAMPGROUND

| HOST SITE | CAMPSITE | PIT TOILETS | PARKING | PICNIC AREA | TRASH | WATER | WASTEWATER DISPOSAL |

TO STEENS MT. LOOP RD. AND FRENCHGLEN

PAY STATION

PUMP HOUSE

DONNER UND BLITZEN RIVER

GETTING THERE

Drive south from just east of Burns on SR 205 about 60 miles to the town of French-glen (named in honor of cattle baron Pete French and his equally ambitious father-in-law, Hugh Glenn). Find North Loop Steens Mountain Road, and head east about 4 miles. The campground is adjacent to the oasis-like Donner and Blitzen River.

GPS COORDINATES

UTM Zone (WGS84) 11T
Easting 0347011
Northing 4740703
Latitude N 42.8036°
Longitude W 118.871°

upland game birds, fur-bearers, and big game. Because Page Springs is open all year, bird enthusiasts should try to plan their trips to the refuge anytime from late February through May, when wave after wave of migratory winged creatures take to the skies: tundra swans, Canada geese, lesser sandhill cranes in February; shorebirds such as willets, long-billed curlews, and avocets in April; and thousands upon thousands of songbirds in May. Beware, however, of the heavy mosquito population present until midsummer. Herds of the wild Kiger mustang, a direct descendant of the horse introduced to America by Spanish conquistadors, still roam areas around the Steens and are managed by the BLM. A wild horse and burro adoption program is a popular and humane means through which the Burns BLM controls the size of these herds.

22
STRAWBERRY
CAMPGROUND

SUMMER TRAVEL IN AND AROUND the historic burgs of Prairie City, John Day, Mount Vernon, Dayville, and Austin is marked by intensely hot days that can sap the strength and resolve of even the hardiest road warrior. If you are about to reach the wilting stage when passing through Prairie City, turn south onto Bridge Street, cross the John Day River, and follow Strawberry Road to its end. Your reward is a cool haven in Malheur National Forest high above the valley floor.

According to a great book called *Oregon Geographical Names,* some of the original settlers named Strawberry Mountain for the abundance of local wild strawberries, and the name just kind of spread to, well, darn near everything else.

Thus, Strawberry Campground is at the end of Strawberry Road, where Strawberry Creek rumbles off of Strawberry Mountain, which is the high point (9,038 feet) of the Strawberry Range and constitutes the focal point of the Strawberry Mountain Wilderness. Oh, yes, there's Strawberry Lake, too. At least it's easy to remember the names of things around here. There's also Strawberry Falls, and I'm sure it's only a matter of time before someone dubs Strawberry Spring!

The drive up to the campground rises gradually through the grassy meadows of private ranchlands and then turns immediately uphill for a gutsy, gravelly climb in the last few miles. As you enter the campground, cross Strawberry Creek to find yourself in a pleasant little forested park hugging the hillside.

The campground is shaped in a near-perfect circle and follows the natural contours of the hillside, with some sites on higher ground, some recessed from the camp road, and some nestled in little glens. It's hard to name the better sites, as most are visible to each other. I suppose the sites on the outer arc of the circle afford

> *Strawberry is a strategically placed, cool wayside stopover when traveling on US 26 through the broad, fascinating plain of the Upper John Day River.*

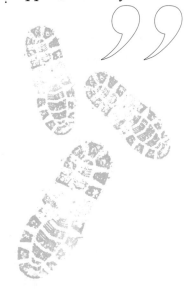

RATINGS

Beauty: ✩ ✩ ✩ ✩
Privacy: ✩ ✩ ✩ ✩
Spaciousness: ✩ ✩ ✩ ✩
Quiet: ✩ ✩ ✩ ✩ ✩
Security: ✩ ✩ ✩
Cleanliness: ✩ ✩ ✩
Insect control: ✩ ✩ ✩

KEY INFORMATION

ADDRESS: Strawberry Campground c/o Prairie City Ranger District P.O. Box 337 Prairie City, OR 97759

OPERATED BY: Malheur National Forest

INFORMATION: (541) 820-3800

OPEN: Late May–October

SITES: 11

EACH SITE: Picnic table, fire grill; shade trees

ASSIGNMENT: First come, first served; no reservations

REGISTRATION: Self-registration on site

FACILITIES: Vault toilets, piped water

PARKING: At campsites

FEE: $8

ELEVATION: 5,700 feet

RESTRICTIONS: *Pets:* On leash only *Fires:* In fire pits only *Alcohol:* Permitted *Vehicles:* RVs and trailers not recommended, no hookups

the most privacy. When I was there, it seemed as though the inner circle of sites was in the process of creating a true inner circle as an afternoon sing-along (a.k.a. party), complete with guitar strumming, shaped up. This might be commonplace given the generally friendly camping atmosphere at Strawberry.

Strawberry Campground is a logical base for some good hiking in the Strawberry Mountain Wilderness, but the elevation gains coming in from the north can be abrupt. A popular route is the Strawberry Basin Trail, which leads to a vista below the summit of Strawberry Mountain. The rise is moderate and the one-way mileage is just over 5 miles, with stops at Strawberry Lake and Strawberry Falls at roughly the 1- and 2-mile marks, respectively. These make for good, short outbound destinations to test the limbs and get the muscles warmed.

Other hiking options await in the Aldrich Mountains to the west and at Lookout Mountain to the east. Access to these two areas requires driving part (or all, if time allows) of the scenic loop that encircles the compact Strawberry Mountain Wilderness. The route is an easy 75 miles, linking two state highways, forest service roads, and a county road—paved the entire way—for a 360-degree view of Grant County's tallest peak and the surrounding environs. Some of the easiest hiking access to Strawberry Mountain's summit is from the south up through Logan Valley. Forest Road 1640 takes you to trailheads that begin deep in a narrow notch between wilderness boundaries, thus putting you within a reasonably short and gradual ascent to the top.

While the pioneers who first made their way into the Upper John Day Basin are long gone, a proud heritage is strongly evident today in the number of historical societies, museums, and markers that preserve the colorful past shaped mainly by the gold mining, ranching, lumbering, and transportation industries. If you're as interested as I am in the human activities that shaped the many fascinating regions of Oregon, take time to visit places such as the Kam Wah Chung & Co. Museum in John Day or the Dewitt Museum in Prairie City. Much can be learned from the artifacts, memorabilia, and photographs on display.

MAP

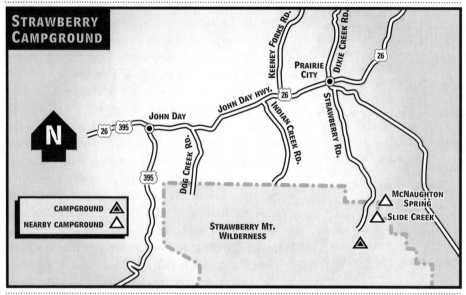

STRAWBERRY CAMPGROUND

KEENEY FORKS RD.
DIXIE CREEK RD.
26
PRAIRIE CITY
JOHN DAY HWY.
26
INDIAN CREEK RD.
STRAWBERRY RD.
JOHN DAY
26 395
DOG CREEK RD.
395
McNAUGHTON SPRING
SLIDE CREEK

CAMPGROUND △
NEARBY CAMPGROUND △

STRAWBERRY MT. WILDERNESS

For a taste of a real working ranch, stop in at Oxbow Ranch on Strawberry Road. The 7,000-square-foot remodeled ranch house operates as a bed-and-breakfast with beautifully appointed guest rooms. For guests of the ranch or out-of-towners passing through, trail-riding and carriage tours are also available (for a fee).

GETTING THERE

From Prairie City, drive south on Strawberry Road for 11 miles to the campground at the road's end. The last several miles climb very steeply and are not recommended for trailers or RVs.

GPS COORDINATES

UTM Zone (WGS84)	11T
Easting	0366431
Northing	4908724
Latitude	N 44.3195°
Longitude	W 118.675°

Lostine

> *Two Pan Campground affords one of the best jumping-off spots for extended backpacking in "America's Little Switzerland."*

TUCKED AWAY IN THE FAR northeastern corner of Oregon on a broad, grassy plain that once was the beloved homeland of the proud Nez Perce Indians sits a magical little kingdom of imposing granite peaks, flower-choked meadows, rushing glacial creeks, and crystalline alpine air.

Eagle Cap Wilderness, rising high above the Wallowa Valley in the Wallowa Mountains, is regularly referred to as "America's Little Switzerland" and even sports a Matterhorn of its own. The American version, which is in a different drainage from our campground, is the second-highest peak in the Wallowas at 9,826 feet; the highest peak is Sacajawea at 9,832 feet.

Following close on their heels, are several dozen peaks above 8,000 feet. In fact, Oregon has 29 peaks that are 9,000 feet or higher. Seventeen of them are clustered in Eagle Cap, the largest wilderness tract in Oregon at more than 350,000 acres.

One of the higher peaks (Eagle Cap, at 9,595 feet) is accessed by a hiking trail right out of Two Pan; the trail leads hikers to the top, so consider picking up a trail map and going for it.

Two Pan Campground may not win any beauty awards on its own, but it is conveniently situated at the intersection of road's end and trail's start, which makes it an ideal base camp for exploring the aforementioned magic kingdom.

The road to Two Pan is also a treat; it follows the Wild and Scenic Lostine River and offers the beauty that is perhaps less evident at Two Pan, piercing deep into the Wallowa range and gaining altitude steadily once it enters the canyon. The drive up from the valley floor and into the canyon is an education in both the geology and history of the area. About a million years ago, a large glacier carved out the Lostine River Canyon as it advanced down from the center of the Wallowa

RATINGS

Beauty: ✿ ✿ ✿ ✿ ✿
Privacy: ✿ ✿ ✿
Spaciousness: ✿ ✿ ✿ ✿
Quiet: ✿ ✿ ✿ ✿ ✿
Security: ✿ ✿ ✿ ✿
Cleanliness: ✿ ✿ ✿ ✿ ✿
Insect control: ✿ ✿ (summer) ✿ ✿ ✿ ✿ (off-season)

Mountains. Grass-covered mounds in the lowlands, known as moraines, are rock and soil deposits left by the glacier in its advance-and-melt periods over hundreds of years. Based on the height of the moraines, geologists estimate that ice as thick as 400 feet once covered this area.

Pole Bridge Picnic Area (a bit past the national forest boundary) is the site of an old bridge, constructed entirely of poles, that once crossed the river here. About all that's left is a piece of foundation, but it's a nice excuse to stop. Fortify yourself for the remainder of the drive with a snack as you examine further evidence of glacial activity in the deep gorge that the river has cut into the canyon. This is about half a mile up the road from the picnic grounds.

Two miles farther is an even better opportunity to view the natural beauty of the Wild and Scenic Lostine River. A short trail takes you to an overlook of Lostine Gorge, a dramatic plunge between steep canyon walls where vegetation works hard to survive amid the predominant rocks and boulders.

The Wallowa Mountains were once the site of busy gold and silver mining. The ramshackle remains of cabins and outbuildings on the privately held Lapover Ranch (at mile 16) are all that remains of mining claims established by settlers from Kansas in 1911. They got in just under the wire—the Wallowa National Forest received its federal designation later that same year. Until Lostine Road was completed to its current end at Two Pan in 1955, the canyon was a popular route for sheepherders moving their flocks to and from the alpine meadows. Apparently, that is how Two Pan got its name—at some point in all their comings and goings, sheepherders passing through left two frying pans hanging from a tree. Okay, not the juiciest story, but facts are facts!

When out sightseeing, you'll be tempted to drink straight from the cold, gushing Lostine to quench your thirst. Hold that thought and keep in mind that the Eagle Cap Wilderness is full of mountain goats, bighorn sheep, elk, deer, and a variety of smaller wild animals. This dramatically increases the risk of giardiasis (a.k.a.

KEY INFORMATION

ADDRESS: Two Pan Campground c/o Eagle Cap Ranger District P.O. Box 907 Baker, OR 97814

OPERATED BY: Wallowa-Whitman National Forest

INFORMATION: (541) 426-5546 Wallowa Mountains Visitors Center

OPEN: Mid-June– November

SITES: 6

EACH SITE: Picnic table, fire grill

ASSIGNMENT: First come, first served; no reservations

REGISTRATION: Not necessary

FACILITIES: Vault toilets, no piped water; stock watering tank and hitch rack

PARKING: In campground

FEE: None

ELEVATION: 5,600 feet

RESTRICTIONS: *Pets:* On leash only *Fires:* In fire pits only *Alcohol:* Permitted *Vehicles:* No RV or trailer accommodations

MAP

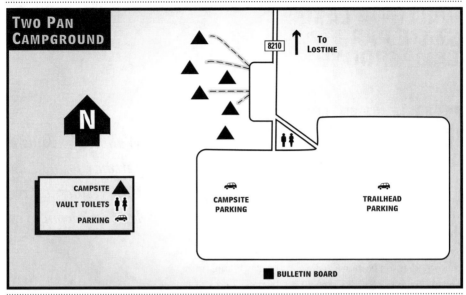

GETTING THERE

To reach Two Pan from Lostine (10 miles west of Enterprise on SR 82), follow Lostine River Road due south all the way to its end at the campground (17 miles). Lostine River Road becomes FS 8250 at the national forest boundary, about halfway to the campground. The road is paved for the first 7 miles out of town.

GPS COORDINATES

UTM Zone (WGS84)   11T
Easting   0470416
Northing   5010848
Latitude   N 45.2505°
Longitude   W 117.377°

diarrhea). Better to boil or treat the glacial flow, unfortunate as that may seem.

If you want seclusion on your exploration of Eagle Cap Wilderness, avoid the Lakes Basin region, which gets overrun by the crowds from Wallowa Lake. If you want to avoid the mosquitoes and biting flies (which are as thick as the crowds in midsummer), go in September. Either way, you'll need a Northwest Forest Pass to park at the trailhead. If you want to treat yourself after roughing it in the wilds, stop in at Wallowa Lake Lodge (on the south shore at the end of SR 82). This fine old resort offers pleasant rooms, fine dining, and lively banter with the friendly staff.

24
WALLOWA LAKE STATE PARK CAMPGROUND

THIS IS THE BIG TAMALE of Oregon campgrounds. It's not really the campground itself that is noteworthy but its impressive neighbors, which set Wallowa Lake State Park apart and make this area a must-visit place. For starters, Wallowa Lake is popular for boating and fishing. Word to the wise: Bring your camera along to snap shots of the sparkling lake surrounded by the snow-capped mountain peaks.

The Wallowa (pronounced Wa-LA-wa) area is also renowned as the entrance point for popular hiking trails and perhaps one of the area's best backpacking trails: the Lakes Basin Trail, where alpine lakes reflect an upclose view of the 10,000-foot peaks of Eagle Cap Wilderness. Simply the drive in will take your breath away as you encounter what are known as the Alps of Oregon. Not to be outdone, Hell's Canyon on the Oregon–Idaho border—a short 30-minute drive away—is the deepest gorge in North America at one mile, and is a popular whitewater-rafting destination.

But you don't need to travel far to see any action. It seems like everything you could possibly want is in this area (including a wedding chapel!). Guided horseback tours, canoeing, restaurants, even bumper cars, and a mini-golf course are among the offerings.

You can also ride a tramway to the top of 8,200-foot Mount Howard, with views of Wallowa Lake and the Eagle Cap Wilderness. Board the tram at quaint Wallowa Lake Village, a town designed to resemble those you might ramble through in the Swiss Alps (it bills itself as "The Switzerland of America").

The little town of Joseph nearby is worth a trip, with local artist galleries and shops lining the main drag. In a world of overdeveloped mountain towns, Joseph is a refreshing blend of modernity that still manages to maintain its authenticity. All of this means one thing, though: it can get packed, especially on a holiday

> *Wallowa Lake is the gateway to the Eagle Cap Wilderness and Hell's Canyon area.*

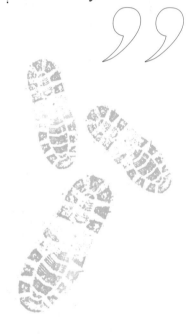

RATINGS

Beauty: ☆ ☆ ☆ ☆ ☆
Privacy: ☆ ☆
Spaciousness: ☆ ☆ ☆
Quiet: ☆ ☆
Security: ☆ ☆ ☆
Cleanliness: ☆ ☆ ☆
Insect control: ☆ ☆ ☆

KEY INFORMATION

ADDRESS: Wallowa Lake State Park
72214 Marina Lane
Joseph, OR 97846

OPERATED BY: Oregon State Parks

INFORMATION: (541) 432-4185, (800) 452-5687; www.oregon stateparks.org

OPEN: Year-round

SITES: 89 tent sites

EACH SITE: Picnic table, fire ring

ASSIGNMENT: First-come, first-served or by reservation at (800) 452-5687 or www .reserveamerica .com ($6 fee)

REGISTRATION: At campground entrance

FACILITIES: Flush toilets, hot showers, laundry, firewood

PARKING: At park entrance and at individual sites

FEE: $13 October–April, $17 May–September; $5 per additional vehicle

ELEVATION: 4,450 feet

RESTRICTIONS: *Pets:* On leash only
Fires: In fire rings only
Alcohol: Permitted at campsites only
Vehicles: RVs and trailers allowed

weekend. (Trust me, you shouldn't even think about showing up without reservations in hand on a long summer weekend unless you want the campground entrance staff to snicker at you).

Besides the campground's 89 tent-only sites, the park offers 121 full-hookup sites, two wooden yurts, and one deluxe two-story cabin.

Bird-watching enthusiasts enjoy Wallowa Lake State Park for the abundance of feathered species that enjoy this lovely land, including pheasants, quail, hummingbirds, and the rarely spotted belted kingfisher. Some of the better birding areas nearby the park include the Chief Joseph Mountain trail and Old Chief Joseph's gravesite.

Guided hunting trips are also popular here; those with the proper permits can pull in big game such as elk, bears, cougars, and even big-horn sheep.

The park offers two picnic areas, a marina, and a boat launch. For those in the mood to test the water, but not necessarily looking to plunge in, try parasailing, offered from May to September. Purchase tickets at the Eagle Cap Packstation.

The Wallowa Lake Highway Forest State Scenic Corridor, a day-use site located along the Wallowa River, is a popular fishing and wildlife-viewing area. Steelhead fishing is popular during the spring and fall. The canyon rises steeply on both sides of the road, and you can almost expect to see deer, elk, and bear that live here. Flowers blanket the area in the spring.

If you come at the end of September, you'll enjoy joining the locals at the town's annual Alpenfest fair, a Swiss-Bavarian festival that has been staged in the traditional Oktoberfest style every autumn since 1974.

If you're looking for a place to bring a group with varied interests—and particularly if you can manage to get away when it's not one of the summer holiday weekends—you can't go wrong with this fascinating area.

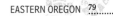

MAP

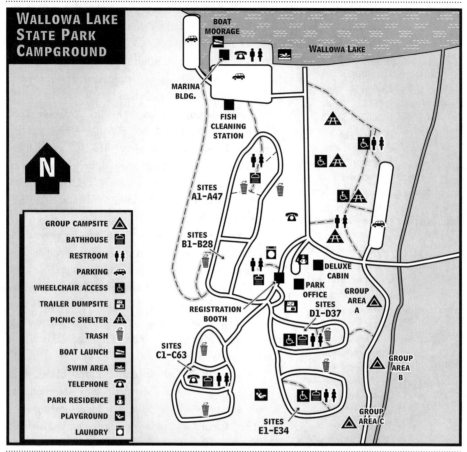

GPS COORDINATES

UTM Zone (WGS84)	11T
Easting	0483765
Northing	5014165
Latitude	N 45.2808°
Longitude	W 117.207°

GETTING THERE

From Enterprise (east of La Grande), drive 12.4 miles south on OR 82 (passing through Joseph) to Wallowa Lake State Park. Continue past Wallowa Lake and turn right into the campground.

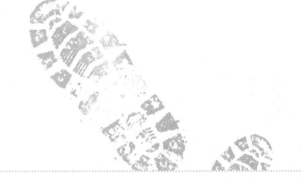

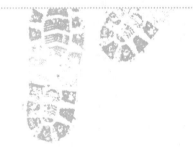

NORTHERN **CASCADES**

25
BADGER LAKE
CAMPGROUND

OKAY. CALL ME A MASOCHIST IF YOU WANT. Perhaps you haven't read enough of this book to know it, but I havfe to come clean with you on one count: I seem to have a perverse penchant for out-of-the-way campgrounds, some of which nearly require being dropped from above.

Well, Badger Lake Campground is no exception. The last stretch of Forest Road 140 (the third forest road you must navigate) is intended only for high-clearance vehicles. Note that I say "intended." If you drove to Badger Lake right now, you would find normal, low-clearance passenger cars parked there. I don't know how they get there. One of these days, I'm going to ask an intrepid driver. Check for wings, maybe. You certainly can't blame campers who put forth the effort. The campground accommodates tent campers only, many of whom revel in the noticeable lack of RVs. (Please don't tell if an RV manages to make the trip when you visit).

Once upon a time, Badger Lake was accessible only by a steep hike up from a trailhead on SR 35. I'm not entirely sure why (or if) the Forest Service considers its road access an improvement over the trail. You may wonder the same thing as you navigate the rough 10 miles on Forest Service roads from the turnoff at Bennett Pass. A good map may keep you from heading off course onto even worse roads (unimaginable!) but won't help much with the road conditions. Pick up the maps you need at the ranger station in Mount Hood on SR 35 south of Hood River. If you are arriving from the east via the Tygh Valley Road, stop at the Barlow Ranger Station in Dufur for information.

It's a good idea to bring along trail maps too, as area hiking is world-class and the only way to enjoy the rugged scenic beauty of this area. The campground itself sits on the northeast edge of Badger Lake in a nonwilderness corridor adjacent to Badger Creek Wil-

> *Hard to get to and even then accessible only in a high-clearance vehicle, the dramatic beauty of Badger Lake is worth the trouble.*

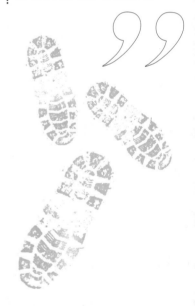

RATINGS

Beauty: ✿ ✿ ✿ ✿ ✿
Privacy: ✿ ✿ ✿
Spaciousness: ✿ ✿ ✿
Quiet: ✿ ✿ ✿ (summer)
✿ ✿ ✿ ✿ ✿ (winter)
Security: ✿ ✿ ✿ ✿ ✿
Cleanliness: ✿ ✿ ✿
Insect control: ✿ ✿

ADDRESS:	Badger Lake Campground c/o Barlow Ranger District 780 NE Court Street Dufur, OR 97021
OPERATED BY:	Mount Hood National Forest
INFORMATION:	(541) 467-2291
OPEN:	July–September
SITES:	4 designated sites; dispersed camping around lake
EACH SITE:	Picnic table, fire grill; shade trees
ASSIGNMENT:	First come, first served; no reservations
REGISTRATION:	Self-registration on site
FACILITIES:	Pit toilets, no piped water
PARKING:	At campsites
FEE:	$10 to camp; Northwest Forest Pass ($5 per day or $30 annually) covers parking at trailhead and day-use only
ELEVATION:	4,472 feet
RESTRICTIONS:	*Pets:* On leash only *Fires:* In fire pits only *Alcohol:* Permitted *Vehicles:* No RVs or trailers, high-clearance vehicles recommended; nonmotorized boats only

derness. This is one of Oregon's smaller designated wilderness areas, with only 26,000 acres. But within this tiny (by western protected-land standards) plot are geographic transitions and climatic changes of dramatic proportions unlike those found in any other comparably sized stretch of Oregon topography.

In this unique microcosm, forested mountains meet dusty lowlands across a span of only 12 miles, with nearly 70 inches of precipitation falling annually on the western ridges but only 20 inches in the eastern sector. Old-growth Douglas firs are gradually replaced by the unusual commingling of ponderosa pine and white oak. For some unexplicable reason, these two tree types are found together only in brief stretches along the Columbia River in Washington and along the same longitudinal line between the Hood River and the Dalles in Oregon. Other arboreal examples of the concentrated, transitional diversity are mountain hemlock, lodgepole pine, and Pacific silver fir. Wildlife includes an Audubon count of 150 bird species, as well as deer and elk sightings.

For the best views of this remarkable landscapes (as well as vistas of mighty Mount Hood), hike to the top of 6,525-foot Lookout Mountain. Numerous other trails lead into the backcountry to such destinations as Gumjuwac Saddle, Gunsight Butte, and Flag Point. The Divide Trail between Lookout Mountain and Flag Point looks down on the canyons of Badger Creek for glimpses of dramatic cliffs and rock formations. Wildflowers such as penstemon, Indian paintbrush, and avalanche lily are at their prime in the eastern portion of the wilderness from spring until late July, at which time the colorful displays jump to higher elevations in the west. In total, roughly 80 miles of trails traverse Badger Creek Wilderness, with connecting routes into Mount Hood Wilderness to the north and west.

Located as it is on the eastern slopes of the Cascades at 4,472 feet, Badger Lake and its adjacent trails are usually not snow free until mid-June but stay clear at least through mid-September. Although heavy snow prohibits travel into this high country in winter, Nordic skiers can take advantage of plowed roads from Bennett Pass southeast toward the wilderness boundary. SR 35

MAP

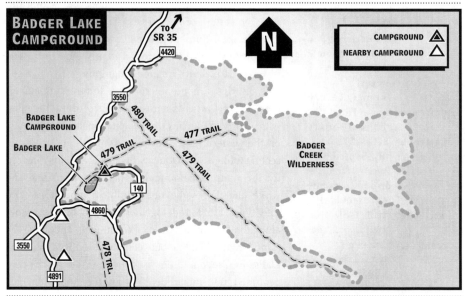

TO
SR 35

4420

N

CAMPGROUND ⛺
NEARBY CAMPGROUND ⛺

3550

480 TRAIL

477 TRAIL

BADGER LAKE
CAMPGROUND

479 TRAIL

BADGER LAKE

479 TRAIL

BADGER
CREEK
WILDERNESS

140

4860

3550

478 TRL.

4891

is kept open all winter to accommodate alpine skiers heading for Mount Hood. Boating on Badger Lake is possible if you didn't lose your canoes on the way in. There's also good rainbow- and brook-trout fishing. The White River Paddle Route farther south along the old Barlow Road (formerly a wagon route for settlers) is another boating option.

The true beauty of Badger Lake Campground is that this remote High Cascade gem really is quite a short drive from metropolitan Portland, making it an easy weekend escape. In less than three hours (factoring in the slowdown on rough roads), you can enjoy a lakeside dinner on a balmy summer evening as you watch the sun sink behind Mount Hood.

GETTING THERE

From the town of Mount Hood (14 miles south of Hood River), travel south on SR 35 for approximately 20 miles to FS 3550. Turn left, and at about 6 miles, turn left onto FS 4860. In 2 miles, turn left again onto FS 140, and follow it to the campground.

GPS COORDINATES

UTM Zone (WGS84)	10T
Easting	0613051
Northing	5017600
Latitude	N 45.3028°
Longitude	W 121.558°

> *This is bare-bones camping at its best: the sky, the sand, the river, and thee. What more could you wish?*

PRIMITIVE. **D**ESOLATE. **R**UGGED. **W**ILD. Haunting. These are a few of the adjectives that quickly come to mind when I think back to my first impressions of Deschutes River country. "Riviere des Chutes" (River of the Falls), as it was originally named by French trappers for the Hudson Bay Company, is the hallowed waterway of central Oregon's high desert.

Flowing north out of Lava Lake just south of Mount Bachelor, the Deschutes (pronounced de shoots) travels toward its confluence with the mighty Columbia River under the protective aegis of state and federal legislation. This is Oregon's second longest river, and its remarkable transformation from docile beginnings above Wickiup Reservoir to a thundering torrent downstream has prompted the separate designations of Upper Deschutes and Lower Deschutes.

Upper Deschutes (from the headwaters to Bend) has been honored with inclusion in the Oregon Scenic Waterway Program for its picturesque, recreational, and natural qualities. Its subtle charms are often overshadowed, however, by its tempestuous lower half, which is the focus of this campground.

The Lower Deschutes River, by far the more popular of the two sections, came under "Wild and Scenic" River protection in 1988. Its untamed whitewater, steep basalt canyon walls, native trout and steelhead, and historic intrigue attract an eclectic array of recreational users from near and far. The "Wild and Scenic" status is the river's best insurance that its unspoiled existence will continue indefinitely for all to enjoy.

Today, Beavertail Campground is one of several minimally developed sites along the eastern bank of the Lower Deschutes that are provided in classic Bureau of Land Management style. You've heard the phrase, "less is more?" It could easily be the BLM motto.

RATINGS

Beauty: ✿ ✿ ✿ ✿ ✿
Privacy: ✿ ✿ ✿
Spaciousness: ✿ ✿ ✿
Quiet: ✿ ✿ ✿ (summer)
✿ ✿ ✿ ✿ ✿ (winter)
Security: ✿ ✿ ✿ ✿ ✿
Cleanliness: ✿ ✿ ✿
Insect control: ✿ ✿

The Bureau knew what it was doing when it created Beavertail. Views across the water from the riverside compound encompass some of the Lower Deschutes' most spectacular basalt canyon walls. Cedar Island is just downstream, so named for a misplaced stand of incense cedar, which typically grows farther west in the Cascades. Wildlife abounds in this area. Be sure to keep your eyes peeled for osprey, river otters, and big horn sheep along the bands of cliffs. So photographers, grab your gear and find a comfortable spot amongst the shore grasses. The kayaks and rafts will be bobbing around the bend any minute.

Speaking of boating, the 51-mile trip from Maupin to the Columbia via the Deschutes requires a permit (available at local outfitters in central Oregon, or on the web at **www.boaterpass.com**). The BLM Web site is full of information for boaters planning a trip on the Lower Deschutes and uses the word "update" fairly often. This might be a good place to start your trip even before leaving the house. The address is **www.or.blm.gov/prineville.** Follow the "Recreation" links from there. For more experienced boaters, there is one class IV rapid (Oak Springs), as well as many less technical runs for novices.

One rapid is in a class all by itself. It's known as Sherar's Falls (pronounced sheerers), and the classification is class VI. This rapid is a mandatory "portage" for all boaters. The falls are still in use today by members of The Confederated Tribes Warm Springs who dipnet for trout and spawning salmon from rickety platforms that teeter precariously over the raging spillway below. I watched in awe for nearly an hour one day as a veteran pulled up a fish about every 10 minutes and clubbed it senseless with one swift bash of a wooden stick. Lashing the dipnet back into position first, he gutted his catch with lightning speed and carefully packed each in a blanket laden with ice. Except for the ice, this was the same technique practiced for centuries.

The climate in this rugged wildwater backcountry is, as you may have guessed, as extreme as the terrain. Summers can be very hot (in the 90s and 100s), while winters generally drop below freezing. The BLM lands in this area are open all year, so make sure you have all the appropriate emergency supplies depending on your

KEY INFORMATION

ADDRESS: Beavertail Campground c/o BLM Prineville District Office 3050 NE 3rd Street Prineville, OR 97754

OPERATED BY: Bureau of Land Management

INFORMATION: (541) 416-6700

OPEN: Year-round

SITES: 17

EACH SITE: Picnic table, tent area; some shade

ASSIGNMENT: First come, first served; no reservations

REGISTRATION: Self-registration

FACILITIES: Vault toilets, hand-pumped water in summer, garbage service, wheel-chair access, boat launch nearby

PARKING: At campsites

FEE: May 15–September 15, weekend nights $12 including parking for 2 vehicles; all other nights $8; $2 per night for each extra vehicle

ELEVATION: 900 feet

RESTRICTIONS: *Pets:* On leash only *Fires:* Detailed fire and smoking restrictions apply; see www.blm.gov/ or/resources/ recreation/site_ info.php?siteid= 330 for all details. *Alcohol:* Permitted *Vehicles:* Driving on vegetation not allowed *Other:* Boating by permit only

MAP

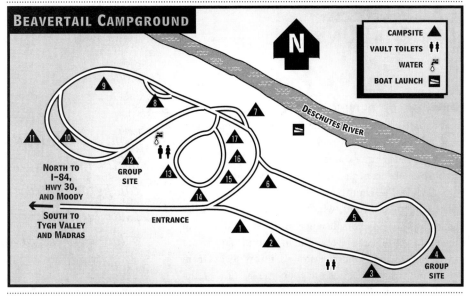

BEAVERTAIL CAMPGROUND

CAMPSITE ▲
VAULT TOILETS ♁♁
WATER ⚱
BOAT LAUNCH ⛵

N

DESCHUTES RIVER

9
8
7
11
10
12
17
16
13
15
6
14

NORTH TO
I-84,
HWY 30,
AND MOODY

GROUP
SITE

SOUTH TO
TYGH VALLEY
AND MADRAS

ENTRANCE

1
2
5
3
4
GROUP
SITE

GETTING THERE

Starting from the eastern side of the (only) bridge in Maupin, drive north about 0.2 miles and turn left onto the Lower Deschutes Access Road. Travel 10 miles until you reach a 3-way stop where the road intersects with OR 216. Turn right (north), and travel 0.75 miles to the first road on your left. Turn left (north) off the pavement and onto the gravel road, which is the continuation of the Lower Deschutes Access Road (large BLM sign here). Follow this gravel road 10 miles to the entrance of Beavertail Campground. Maupin is 42 miles south of The Dalles on US 197.

choice of season. Gusty winds and sudden thunderstorms are commonplace. This is a spare campground with the typical scraggly vegetation of the high desert such as small juniper trees, sagebrush, and native grasses. In other words, there are no towering evergreens to protect you. The car may be the best place to dive if the elements get out of control.

The road that accesses Beavertail and all other BLM dispersed and managed sites is officially known as the Lower Deschutes National Backcountry Byway. But it is commonly labeled Deschutes River Access Road on maps. More information about the scenic byway can be obtained on the **byways.org** Web site. This thoroughfare can be quite crowded in summer, especially on weekends. Use caution if you choose to explore by mountain bike. Gravel goes flying as cars careen past.

GPS COORDINATES

UTM Zone (WGS84)   10T
Easting   660544
Northing   5022375
Latitude   N 45.3365°
Longitude   W 120.951°

27
CAMP CREEK
CAMPGROUND

TIRED OF DRIVING FOREVER on rough forest roads just to find a place to set up camp? Then check out Camp Creek. You can't beat the convenience of this campground, located directly off US 26 right in the heart of the Mount Hood National Forest.

While the campground itself doesn't have supplies (except firewood, which you can buy from the camp host), it's a short distance to the small mountain towns of Zigzag and Government Camp. You won't even realize that you're a stone's throw away from civilization once you set up your tent at one of the creekside sites, which provide white noise as a pleasant, natural backdrop. The shade of the Douglas fir trees and the rushing creek give you the feeling of having gotten away from it all. Although, as with many of the area campgrounds, it tends to get a little crowded. The beauty of Camp Creek Campground is that the sites are relatively spacious, so you won't feel like you're on top of your neighbor. In one of our favorite sites, there is a seat carved out of a tree trunk where you can sit and enjoy a private view of the moon lighting up the creek below. The campground was originally constructed by the Civilian Conservation Corps in 1936. Some features from this era remain, such as several stone fireplaces.

Only 20 miles east of Portland, Mount Hood National Forest totals 1,067,043 acres, of which 189,200 are in designated wilderness areas. Mount Hood Wilderness, the largest area, encompasses the summit and upper slopes of its namesake peak. The forest is laced with hiking trails, many within a few miles of Camp Creek. In fact, the 1.6-mile Still Creek Trail starts in the campground; the Forest Service website describes it as "simply a pleasant forest trail . . . there is a short section of decked trail that goes through a wet cedar grove." Sounds like a nice after-dinner stroll, doesn't it? Fishing, berry-picking, bird-watching, bicycling, and mushroom-hunting are also popular activities in the area.

> *Conveniently located off the highway, this campground is a great place for a quick getaway to the Mount Hood area.*

RATINGS

Beauty: ☆ ☆ ☆ ☆
Privacy: ☆ ☆ ☆
Spaciousness: ☆ ☆ ☆
Quiet: ☆ ☆ ☆
Security: ☆ ☆ ☆
Cleanliness: ☆ ☆ ☆ ☆
Insect control: ☆ ☆ ☆ ☆

KEY INFORMATION

ADDRESS: Camp Creek
Campground
c/o Zigzag Ranger
District
70220 East US 26
Zigzag, OR 97049

OPERATED BY: Mount Hood
National Forest

INFORMATION: (503) 622-3191

OPEN: Mid-April–early
October

SITES: 25

EACH SITE: Picnic table, fire
ring

ASSIGNMENT: First come, first
served or by
reservation at
(877) 444-6777 or
www.recreation
.gov

REGISTRATION: With camp host

FACILITIES: Hand-pumped
water, vault
toilets, firewood
for sale

PARKING: At campsites only

FEE: $16; $8 per additional vehicle

ELEVATION: 2,200 feet

RESTRICTIONS: *Pets:* On leash only
Fires: In fire rings
only
Alcohol: Permitted
at campsites only
Vehicles: 22-foot RV
size limit

Hidden Lake Trail, the longest major trail within Mount Hood Wilderness, departs from a trailhead off FS 2639 (Kiwanis Camp Road), which intersects OR 26 5 miles east of the hamlet of Rhododendron. Along the path you'll spot many of the flowering shrubs for which the town is named (blossoming in profusion in June) as you ascend to a forested lake. A round-trip to the terminus (beyond the lake) totals 10 miles. The easier 0.6-mile Little Zigzag Falls Trail also departs from FS 2639 to follow Little Zigzag Creek to its namesake falls. The best hike in the area is the Mirror Lake Trail, just seven miles up Highway 26; follow it 1.5 miles gradually uphill to a lovely lake with a view of Mount Hood, or go another two miles up to the top of Tom-Dick-Harry Ridge, where the view is astounding. You can get the latest area trail information by visiting **www.mthood .info,** which will give you details on snow conditions, recent trail maintenance, and permit requirements.

The Zigzag Ranger District also sponsors several wildflower hikes during the summer. The popular Top Spur Trail leads through flower-cloaked meadows to the crest of Bald Mountain and then on to McNeil Point, and the Trillium Lake Trail traverses colorful fields at the water's edge. Contact the district at (503) 622-3191 for guided-hike schedules and for additional information on Mount Hood's many trails. Note that trailhead parking requires a Northwest Forest Pass ($5 per day or $30 annually).

If you want close-up view of the 11,237-foot Mount Hood, Oregon's tallest mountain, take the 6-mile winding drive up to historic Timberline Lodge, which sits midway up the summit of the mountain and offers restaurants and hiking trails with a great view of the mountain—and some fine beverages.

Overall, Camp Creek is a great base camp for anything you might want to do in the Mount Hood area, and with its convenience combined with great scenery, it's one of the tops in this popular region. Consequently, you may want to reserve a creekside site if you plan to go on a holiday weekend, or any sunny summer weekend for that matter, as those are the best plots of the bunch.

MAP

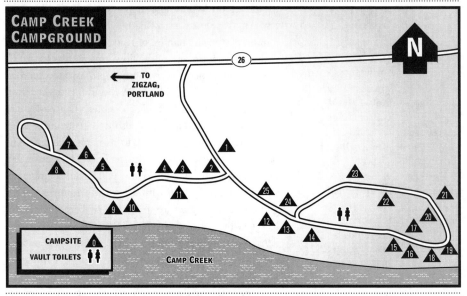

GETTING THERE

From Portland, drive east on
US 26 for 35 miles to Zigzag.
Continue through Zigzag and
drive 4 miles to the campground on the right-hand
side of the highway.

GPS COORDINATES

UTM Zone (WGS84)	10T
Easting	0588272
Northing	5017561
Latitude	N 45.306°
Longitude	W 121.874°

> *If you're cruising along I-84 to Portland beside the Columbia River and you've just about given up on finding a campground not swarming with RVs, all is not lost.*

YES, I KNOW IT'S HARD TO BELIEVE, but the Columbia River Gorge does have a campground that is not overrun with tourists in RVs. And, it has the distinction of being considered the oldest official Forest Service campground in the U.S.

Built in 1915, Eagle Creek Campground is perched above the Columbia River and the very busy I-84 corridor in a rustic setting that has changed little since it first opened. Then, Eagle Creek sported amenities that must have been talked about from Portland to Pendleton: flush toilets that are still in use today!

Eagle Creek is quite a pleasant surprise, whether you plan a sojourn high into the backcountry of the Columbia Wilderness or just need a shady afternoon respite from the freeway below. Situated within the Columbia River Gorge National Scenic Area (headquartered in Hood River 20 miles east), the campground lies just east of the Bonneville Dam almost equidistant between the towns of Bonneville and Cascade Locks. It's easy to miss the turnoff, and it's hard to slow down, too. Everyone drives like a bat out of hell on I-84—except, of course, for the occasional boardhead bound for a little windsurfing in Hood River sputtering along in (you guessed it) a battered Volkswagen minibus.

Once you're off the freeway with car and nerves intact, nose through the lower parking area and follow the camp road up through towering true fir, western red cedar, and hemlock trees to the campground. The busy freeway teeming with tourists and those intractable tractor-trailers will quickly fade into oblivion, if only temporarily. You'll be surprised at how remote you feel in just a few minutes!

Despite this sense of isolation at the campground, if you've come to hike the trails, you probably won't be alone. Trails throughout the Eagle Creek basin and up into the Columbia Wilderness are some of the most

RATINGS

Beauty: ✪ ✪ ✪ ✪
Privacy: ✪ ✪ ✪ ✪
Spaciousness: ✪ ✪ ✪
Quiet: ✪ ✪ ✪ (summer)
✪ ✪ ✪ ✪ ✪ (winter)
Security: ✪ ✪ ✪
Cleanliness: ✪ ✪ ✪ ✪
Insect control: ✪ ✪ ✪

popular in the Columbia River Gorge. But the main trail has many spurs that can be traversed to and fro or combined with other trails to create loop trips. There is a network of trails more than 90 miles within the Columbia Wilderness (including 14 of the Pacific Crest Trail alone), so you're bound to find some solitude if you have time to wander. While there are varying trail lengths to accommodate all skill levels, it should be noted that the preponderance involve respectable elevation gains, with beginning points starting just above sea level and destination lakes, ridges, and plateaus topping out around 4,000 feet.

The historic Eagle Creek Trail, also built in 1915, is an example of a long, gradual ascension; it parallels Eagle Creek for about seven miles, then climbs six miles more up to Wahtum Lake. Along the way, the trail passes high cliffs along Eagle Creek and oodles of waterfalls (Punchbowl Falls being the most notable), then crests atop the broad plateau of Waucoma Ridge, which looks out over the expansive Columbia River Gorge and south to Mount Hood. Ruckel Creek Trail, on the other hand, just east of the campground via a short connector trail, is a rigorous 6-mile climb nearly straight up to Benson Plateau for 3,700 feet of elevation gain.

Two loop trips—one shorter, one ambitious—incorporate stretches of the Pacific Crest Trail, which crosses the Columbia River at the Bridge of the Gods (a worthy sidetrip of its own) and passes through the wilderness to its boundary at Wahtum Lake. Ask park staff for directions and details. For the most accurate picture of the trail system within Columbia Wilderness and to find hikes that suit your comfort level, check with the Mount Hood National Forest headquarters in Sandy.

Weatherwise, this is an area of transition between moisture-laden western Oregon and the more arid climes in the east. The Gorge itself adds its own wind-tunnel effect, so prepare for variety even in summer. Thunderstorms materialize quickly, and the wind can blow hard, particularly in late afternoon. In fact, the Columbia River has achieved an international reputation among sailboarders for this exact reason. The discovery has transformed the burg of Hood River, once a quiet farming and fishing community, into a veritable

KEY INFORMATION

ADDRESS:	Eagle Creek Campground c/o Columbia River Gorge 902 Wasco Ave., Suite 200 Hood River, OR 97031
OPERATED BY:	Columbia River Gorge National Scenic Area
INFORMATION:	(541) 308-1700
OPEN:	Late April– September
SITES:	20
EACH SITE:	Picnic table, fire pit with grill
ASSIGNMENT:	First come, first served; no reservations
REGISTRATION:	Self-registration on site
FACILITIES:	Bathhouse with flush toilets and piped water (no showers)
PARKING:	At campsites
FEE:	$15
ELEVATION:	200 feet
RESTRICTIONS:	*Pets:* On leash only *Fires:* In fire grates only *Alcohol:* Permitted *Vehicles:* 20-foot RV and trailer size limit, no hookups

MAP

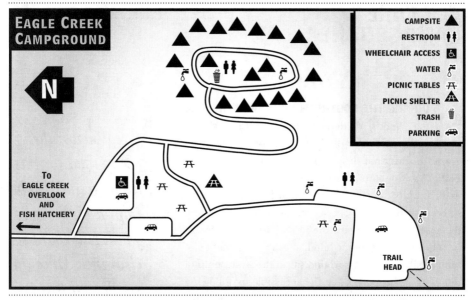

GETTING THERE

From Portland, drive 41 miles east on I-84 to Exit 41 (2 miles past the town of Bonneville). From the east on I-84, there is no westbound exit, so continue 2 miles to Exit 40, Bonnevile Dam, and return to the interstate eastbound to Exit 41. At the stop sign, turn right and follow signs to Eagle Creek. You'll come first to a lower day-use parking area, but continue up the winding road through the forest to the campground.

GPS COORDINATES

UTM Zone (WGS84) 10T
Easting   0584013
Northing   5054549
Latitude   N 45.6394°
Longitude   W 121.922°

Mecca of sailboard mania, with renovated hotels, bed-and-breakfasts, trendy shops, espresso bars, microbreweries, and cafes catering to a transient population that literally comes and goes with the wind.

Long before the windsurfers, Native Americans were the first to pay homage to the winds of the Columbia. Lewis and Clark were the first white explorers to use the river as a highway, opening the door to continued use by settlers who, at The Dalles, traded Conestoga wagons for the steamboats that carried them to their new homes in the Northwest territory. Rapids and falls that had to be portaged then no longer exist today because the wild and mighty flow of the Columbia was harnessed by power companies in the twentieth century.

For those curious about the hydroelectric business and wanting a respite from outdoor activities, the Bonneville Dam gives tours daily. Other points of interest nearby—both indoors and out—include Cascade Locks, Crown Point Vista House and Observatory, Multnomah Falls and Multnomah Falls Lodge, Bridal Veil Falls, and Fort Dalles Museum.

29
ELK LAKE
CAMPGROUND

HUGGING THE SOUTHERN BOUNDARY of Bull of the Woods Wilderness, peaceful Elk Lake is aptly named for the huge herds of elk that once grazed in this area. It lies in the subalpine shadow of Battle Ax Mountain, Mount Beachie, and Gold Butte, and is a classic Cascade escape that probably remains so because the Forest Service insists on not improving the access road. (Perhaps the ill maintenance is intentional, but on the other hand, it may be a matter of funds.) Elk Lake Campground sits at the western tip of this peanut-shaped lake and is accessible by following the road along the north side of the lake to the short spur that drops down off the main road to the left.

Elk Lake's campsites are strung along the shore of the lake. Tall stands of Douglas fir and western hemlock share the land with white fir, birches, Oregon grape, ferns, and trillium to offer a prime collection of natural cover. In early July, pink-blossomed rhododendrons seem somehow out of place in this rugged, woodsy setting.

This campground may be tough to get to, but once you're there, it makes for a terrific base camp while you enjoy the region's recreational options. At the top of the list is hiking into Bull of the Woods Wilderness, which is home to one of western Oregon's few remaining old-growth forests. From Beachie Saddle (about a mile west of the campground on FS 4697), trailheads strike out for Battle Ax Mountain to the north (into the wilderness) and Mount Beachie to the south. This section of FS 4697 is not recommended for any motor vehicles; consider this a warm-up for the steep 2-mile and 1.5-mile grunts up Battle Ax and Beachie, respectively. You will be greeted, however, by views that are well worth the effort. A less strenuous hike follows Elk Lake Creek northeast into Bull of the Woods Wilderness from a trailhead near where the creek feeds

> *Great news: the access road for this campground has been improved, though you'll still want some clearance. Once there, you'll find this is a great base camp for exploring Willamette National Forest and two wilderness areas.*

RATINGS

Beauty: ✿ ✿ ✿ ✿ ✿
Privacy: ✿ ✿ ✿ ✿
Spaciousness: ✿ ✿ ✿ ✿ ✿
Quiet: ✿ ✿ ✿ ✿ ✿
Security: ✿ ✿ ✿
Cleanliness: ✿ ✿ ✿ ✿
Insect Control: ✿ ✿ ✿

KEY INFORMATION

ADDRESS: Elk Lake Campground c/o Detroit Ranger District HC 73, Box 320 Mill City, OR 97360

OPERATED BY: Willamette National Forest

INFORMATION: (503) 854-3366

OPEN: July–late September

SITES: 14

EACH SITE: Picnic table, fire pit with grill; shade trees

ASSIGNMENT: First come, first served; no reservations

REGISTRATION: Not necessary

FACILITIES: Vault toilets, primitive boat launch; no piped water and no garbage service (pack out all garbage)

PARKING: At campsites and in general parking area (a short walk to some campsites); high clearance recommended

FEE: None, though there are plans to implement one for 2009, probably around $12.

ELEVATION: 4,000 feet

RESTRICTIONS: *Pets:* On leash only
Fires: In fire pits only
Alcohol: Permitted
Vehicles: Not recommended for low-clearance vehicles

its namesake. For extended trips into the wilderness backcountry, take the trail that leaves very near the campground spur road. In 1998, a sizeable chunk of Bull of the Woods Wilderness was annexed to help create adjoining Opal Creek Wilderness, so be sure you have a current map of the area showing both areas.

If you are thinking Elk Lake might be a nice spot to take in lazy kayaking or canoeing, you're right. Anyone foolhardy enough to drag a boat into this remote locale deserves to be rewarded (or psychoanalyzed). An undeveloped put-in accommodates inflatable rafts, kayaks, canoes, and other small, nonmotorized craft. Pick up a fishing permit at the general store in Detroit if you have thoughts of angling for your dinner. For either boating or fishing, don't overlook little Dunlap Lake (named for an early prospector), which is hidden from view about a mile before you get to Elk Lake. Forest Service roads also await exploration if you have the foresight to bring your mountain bike along. Test your skill downhill on the 2-mile "riverbed" and pedal on up FS 4696 (to the left) to Gold Butte. The views of mountain peaks from this formerly manned fire lookout are staggering on a clear day—north to Mount Hood, east to Mount Jefferson, south to Mount Washington. Farther up FS 46 is Breitenbush Hot Springs, worth a dip for tired muscles.

MAP

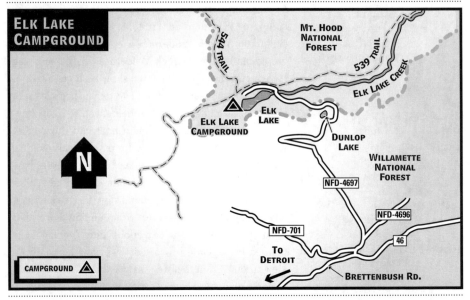

ELK LAKE CAMPGROUND

544 TRAIL

MT. HOOD NATIONAL FOREST

539 TRAIL

ELK LAKE CREEK

N

ELK LAKE CAMPGROUND

ELK LAKE

DUNLOP LAKE

WILLAMETTE NATIONAL FOREST

NFD-4697

NFD-4696

NFD-701

46

TO DETROIT

BRETTENBUSH RD.

CAMPGROUND

GETTING THERE

To reach Elk Lake Campground from Detroit (50 miles southeast of Salem), drive north on FS 46 (Breitenbush Road) 4.5 miles to FS 4697. Turn left and continue 10 miles to the campground. Stay to the left fork where FS 4697 and FS 4696 intersect at about 8 miles.

GPS COORDINATES

UTM Zone (WGS84)	10T
Easting	0571393
Northing	4963307
Latitude	N 44.8196°
Longitude	W 122.097°

30
ELKHORN VALLEY CAMPGROUND

> *This is minimalist camping at its best in a heavily forested compound along the Little North Santiam River.*

I AM NOT AT ALL ASHAMED TO ADMIT that I had an ulterior motive when I was planning to visit Elkhorn Valley Recreation Site. You see, there's this golf course I'd read about . . .

For years, I'd heard about an 18-hole track east of Salem that had gained national recognition for its outstanding natural setting and challenging layout. Being above-average in my passion for the game (there are those who will say crazy), I cleverly crafted an itinerary that put me in the neighborhood. I figured a golf game would be an excellent antidote to the camping overdose and allow me to stretch my road-weary limbs.

I soon discovered that showing up at Elkhorn Valley Golf Course as a single on a brilliant Sunday morning in the summertime is more foolhardy than hoping to find a campground free of RVs.

Sulking back to my car, I was downright irritated to have my perfect plan botched. I sat on the tailgate, drinking cold coffee and eating a stale donut, contemplating my options. I watched enviously as foursome after foursome with tee times pulled into the parking lot, making way too much noise for a breathless summer morning and talking that pre-round talk: "I've got 75 in my bones today, boys, so just give me your money now and it will seem a whole lot less painful later on."

That was enough for me. Off to Elkhorn Valley Recreation Site I went, and what a treat that was! Who needs golf, anyway?

Nestled along the Little North Santiam River under dense stands of old growth, Elkhorn Valley Recreation Site has the feel of a campground much farther removed from the urban pace than one would expect within an easy 33 miles of metropolitan Salem. The North Fork Road in from OR 22 is paved all the way (although there are a surprising number of dips and twists to keep inattentive drivers alert). Within minutes

RATINGS

Beauty: ✿ ✿ ✿ ✿ ✿
Privacy: ✿ ✿ ✿ ✿
Spaciousness: ✿ ✿ ✿ ✿
Quiet: ✿ ✿ ✿ ✿
Security: ✿ ✿ ✿ ✿ ✿
Cleanliness: ✿ ✿ ✿ ✿ ✿
Insect control: ✿ ✿

of the turn to the northeast along the Elkhorn Valley corridor, the weekend escapist is treated to a deep green enclave that immediately soothes the spirit.

Designed in standard minimalist Bureau of Land Management style, Elkhorn Valley has 24 campsites simply staged in three generously-spaced clusters, areas A, B, and D—not sure what happened to C. It's hard to say which area is best; chances are you'll take whatever you can get if it's a busy summer weekend, as availability is first-come, first-served. Area A has the most sites (10) and is situated closest to the North Fork Road. I found these sites to be the most closely spaced. Area D is at the end of the camp road, affording the greatest sense of being tucked into the forest, but this is also a turnaround point for campers heading back out and has the potential for traffic clogs. Sites in Area B are closest to the river and are set up in more of a walk-in fashion.

For the most part, each site and parking space is positioned in such a way so as not to unduly infringe upon neighboring sites. Each comes with picnic table and fire pit. Unlike most compounds of this relatively intimate nature, each cluster has its own pay station and restroom for true self-sufficiency. There's a Rim Trail that runs the entire ridge above the three areas and a River Trail between areas B and D. A spur trail connects the Rim Trail to the River Trail via a handy boardwalk and footbridge elevated above the soggy lowland behind area D.

You don't have to go far to enjoy spectacular scenery in Elkhorn Valley. While the campground's primeval forest setting may be enough for you, a short drive further up the North Fork Road past Elkhorn Valley Golf Course and Shady Cove Campground puts you at the access point for the Opal Creek Wilderness, a fairly recent addition to Oregon's wilderness collection designated in 1998. The Opal Creek Scenic Recreation Area designation came even more recently in 2002.

This small but notable wilderness tract is home to two wild and scenic rivers (Opal Creek and Battle Ax Creek). Just as importantly, it protects some of the last great old-growth trees of the Willamette Valley, with one Douglas fir in particular on the trail to Opal Pool known to be 1,000 years old. It is not uncommon to pass stands

KEY INFORMATION

ADDRESS:	Elkhorn Valley Campground c/o BLM Salem District Office 1717 Fabry Rd. SE Salem, OR 97306
OPERATED BY:	Bureau of Land Management
INFORMATION:	(503) 375-5646
OPEN:	Memorial Day– Labor Day
SITES:	24
EACH SITE:	Picnic table, fire grill; shade
ASSIGNMENT:	First-come, first-served; no reservations
REGISTRATION:	Self-registration on site
FACILITIES:	Vault toilets, potable water, picnic area, firewood for purchase, garbage service, river access, trails, camp host
PARKING:	At campsites; maximum 2 vehicles per site with overflow parking available
FEE:	$10; $5 per additional vehicle
ELEVATION:	1,200 feet
RESTRICTIONS:	*Pets:* On leash only *Fires:* In fire pits *Alcohol:* Permitted *Vehicles:* Large trailers not recommended due to extremely tight turns *Other:* 14-day stay limit; no gathered wood more than 1" in diameter; gate closed 10 p.m.–7 a.m.

MAP

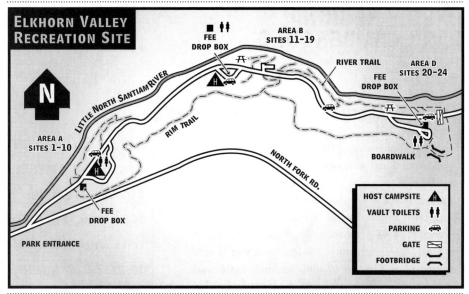

GETTING THERE

From Salem, drive 24 miles east on OR 22 towards Detroit. At Lyons, turn left onto North Fork Road and drive 9 miles to the campground on the left. You'll pass Canyon Creek Day-Use Area on the way.

of trees on various other trails in the Opal Creek Wilderness with specimens easily between 500 and 750 years old. Take your pick of several lowland or highland hikes that also take in views of waterfalls, crystal clear pools, and rugged mountain peaks. The Opal Creek Ancient Forest Center also offers workshops and other events; see **www.opalcreek.org** for more information.

The lands in the Elkhorn Valley corridor are operated under a sometimes-confusing conglomeration of state forest, national forest, and BLM jurisdiction. It's best to contact the BLM or Willamette National Forest for a good overview map of the area.

GPS COORDINATES

UTM Zone (WGS84)   10T
Easting   0542313
Northing   4960761
Latitude   N 44.799°
Longitude   W 122.465°

31
OXBOW REGIONAL PARK CAMPGROUND

I N THE LARGEST CITY in one of the nation's most conservation-minded states, Portland's Oxbow Regional Park sets a prime example of what a metropolitan park can and should be. The grounds are a sprawling 1,000 acres of dense forests, grassy clearings, Sandy River frontage, and sheer canyon walls. Old-growth forest covers 180 acres. Native salmon spawn within one-quarter mile of camping areas on the Sandy River, known as the top-rated winter steelhead stream in Oregon. Wildlife abounds in the park, with more than 200 native plant varieties, 100 bird species, nearly 40 different mammals, and an interesting assortment of reptiles and water-dwelling creatures. The park employs a full-time naturalist year-round, who is busiest in summer thanks to a heavy schedule of public and private programs.

Campers enjoy a choice of more campsites (22 have been added for a total of 67) and two new restrooms, with the ultimate in camping comfort: Flush toilets arrived at Oxbow along with hot showers, heated bathroom floors, and hot-air hand dryers. It's almost better than home—but still with all the other rustic charms and natural beauty that make this such a great park.

You'll have a hard time deciding what to do first, once you've set up camp—and you should do that as soon as you arrive. Sites are first-come, first-served, although it would be hard to find a bad spot. The park staff has been busy improving the privacy between sites with natural vegetation and cedar fences. It's music to the ears of tent campers everywhere when peace and quiet become a priority.

The first order of business after finding your spot may be to explore the trails on foot. There are roughly 15 miles of trail that follow the Sandy River and wind throughout the park. It's easy to lose yourself in the spaciousness and ramble to your heart's content with no

> *An easy 20 miles from downtown Portland, Oxbow Regional Park is an amazing blend of recreational diversity, scenic delight, and environmental consciousness.*

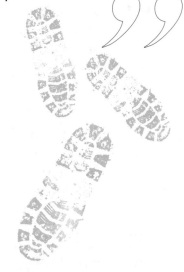

RATINGS

Beauty: ✿ ✿ ✿ ✿ ✿
Privacy: ✿ ✿ ✿ ✿
Spaciousness: ✿ ✿ ✿ ✿
Quiet: ✿ ✿ ✿ ✿
Security: ✿ ✿ ✿ ✿ ✿
Cleanliness: ✿ ✿ ✿ ✿
Insect control: ✿ ✿ ✿ ✿

KEY INFORMATION

ADDRESS: Oxbow Regional Park
3010 SE Oxbow Parkway
Gresham, OR 97080

OPERATED BY: Metro

INFORMATION: (503) 663-4708

OPEN: All year; gates close at sunset and open at 6:30 a.m.

SITES: 67 total (12 for RVs)

EACH SITE: Picnic table, free-standing barbecue grill, lantern pole, shade trees

ASSIGNMENT: First come, first served; no reservations

REGISTRATION: Daily fee collected each evening at campsite; vehicle fee at entrance

FACILITIES: Flush toilets, hot showers, heated restroom floors; firewood for sale, group camps, playground, boat ramp, equestrian area, interpretive programs

PARKING: At campsites (2 vehicles max)

FEE: $15; $4 per vehicle fee

ELEVATION: Sea level

RESTRICTIONS: *Pets:* Not permitted
Fires: In fire pits only, subject to seasonal restrictions
Alcohol: Not allowed
Vehicles: 35-foot RV size limit, no hookups; no ATVs
Other: No guns or fireworks; no gathering firewood

other thought than to see how many of the birds on the park's list (available at the office) you can identify. Wander into the old-growth forest and contemplate a summer idyll. There's a small waterfall nearby to enhance your poetic musings. Slip through the underbrush to a sun-warmed curve in the river and wriggle your toes in the sand. Even at the height of the summer season, you'll be amazed at how quickly you can find seclusion.

For a different perspective of the trail system, the park allows horses on most of the pathways. There are designated equestrian unloading areas, and trailhead markers indicate those that are restricted.

Fishing and boating activities are undeniably central to the popularity of Oxbow Park and Sandy River. Most often they go hand in hand. There are very few times of the year when anglers won't find a reason to cast their lines into the broad and shallow waters. Along with its preeminent status as a steelheader's delight, the Sandy also sports healthy quantities of coho, fall and spring chinook, and summer steelhead. Check with the park office for fishing regulations on the Sandy, as they differ from those of other Oregon rivers.

Recreational boating on this section of the Sandy is limited to nonmotorized craft, thanks to the recent state and federal designations of the "Wild and Scenic" Sandy River. Above Oxbow Park, and dependent on flow levels, there is Class III and IV whitewater for experienced kayakers, rafters, and canoeists to enjoy. A popular run is the 6 miles between Dodge Park and Oxbow, affording exclusive views of this section of the river gorge. Downstream from Oxbow to Lewis and Clark State Park is a pleasant drift trip with gentle ripples and refreshing pools for an occasional dip. Additional river and boat-rental information is available at the park office.

If you're interested in exploring beyond the park's boundaries, Oxbow can be the starting point for a couple of scenic drives that allow you to see a lot with minimal time commitments. The shorter of the two is the route along Crown Point Highway, named for the 700-foot piece of basalt that spires above the Columbia River. Crown Point Vista House, with its information center, is well worth the visit, not to mention the staggering views afforded from its lofty perch.

MAP

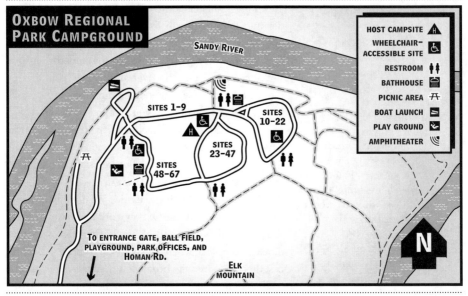

OXBOW REGIONAL PARK CAMPGROUND

SANDY RIVER

SITES 1-9

SITES 10-22

SITES 23-47

SITES 48-67

HOST CAMPSITE	H
WHEELCHAIR-ACCESSIBLE SITE	♿
RESTROOM	🚻
BATHHOUSE	
PICNIC AREA	🏕
BOAT LAUNCH	
PLAY GROUND	
AMPHITHEATER	

TO ENTRANCE GATE, BALL FIELD, PLAYGROUND, PARK OFFICES, AND HOMAN RD.

ELK MOUNTAIN

N

The second route takes you southeast on US 26 through the Sandy River lowlands, around Mount Hood, north to Hood River on SR 35, and back along I-84 to Exit 18 at Lewis and Clark State Park. This is roughly 150 miles of non-stop scenery, with the snowy peak of Mount Hood as the focal point most of the way. From Hood River back to Oxbow, the changing landscape of the Columbia River Gorge unfolds around each bend in the road.

Oxbow is a well-managed park that gives foremost consideration to the interests of its visitors. There is even a ranger on duty in the park 24 hours per day in the event of an emergency.

GETTING THERE

To reach Oxbow Park, take Exit 16, Wood Village, off I-84 in Gresham. Go south to Division Street. Turn left, and continue to Oxbow Parkway. From there, follow signs down to the park. The road winds around a bit, and there are several spots where it is easy to make a miscalculated turn. Just keep following the signs. Once you reach the park entrance, it's a sharp and curving drop down into the gorge.

GPS COORDINATES

UTM Zone (WGS84)   10T
Easting   0555395
Northing   5038430
Latitude   N 45.4972°
Longitude   W 122.291°

32
SILVER FALLS
STATE PARK
CAMPGROUND

Oregon's largest state park is a destination in itself, with everything from horseback riding to waterfalls to hiking trails on its premises.

IF YOU'RE LOOKING FOR A WEEKEND destination where you can see it all in one place, Silver Falls State Park is the place to go. As the largest state park in Oregon, the 8,700-acre Silver Falls is renowned for its hiking. The 7-mile Silver Creek Canyon Trail (also known as Trail of Ten Falls) traverses a lush forest floor covered with Oregon grape, salal, and sword ferns beneath second-growth fir, hemlock, and cedar trees.

The trail follows the north and south forks of Silver Creek, passing 10 waterfalls en route. It runs behind several tall falls and along the edges of others. Bring your camera along for the South Falls, the largest of the falls, which plummets 177 feet and backs up to a tunnel through which visitors can view the cascade. If you feel like you've seen it before, you probably have, as Silver Falls is one of the most-photographed places in the state. Hiking the entire circuit can take at least three hours, so pack a picnic lunch and make an all-day excursion of it. To preserve its primitive nature, the trail is uninterrupted by picnic tables, shelters, or restrooms.

If you want to let someone else do the walking, horse rentals are also a popular activity in this park, where you can arrange one-hour guided tours. The park includes more than 25 miles of hiking trails, 14 miles of horse trails, plus several biking paths, so there will be plenty to keep you busy (make sure to get a handy map at the park entrance). Wildlife you may spot while on the trail includes blacktail deer, black bears, and cougars, although beavers and chipmunks are more likely.

If you feel like taking a dip, there is a developed beach on the east shore of Silver Creek. There is no lifeguard on duty; restrooms, a snack bar, and a playground are located nearby.

Silver Falls State Park took its name from the former town of Silver Falls City, population 200, which stood where the South Falls parking lot now lies. (It

RATINGS

Beauty: ✿ ✿ ✿
Privacy: ✿ ✿ ✿
Spaciousness: ✿ ✿ ✿
Quiet: ✿ ✿ ✿
Security: ✿ ✿ ✿ ✿
Cleanliness: ✿ ✿ ✿ ✿
Insect control: ✿ ✿ ✿

officially became a park in the early 1930s.) Evidence of the town's main source of income—logging—remains in some of the park's large cedar stumps—notches from springboards the loggers wedged into the trees' trunks to cut them. At the historic South Falls Lodge, you can enjoy a post-hike latté and take a glimpse back into history through the collection of old logging photos and antique tools. The lodge, originally designed as a restaurant, was constructed by the Civilian Conservation Corps and Works Project Administration in the 1930s, closed in the late 1950s, and restored pursuant to its placement on the National Register of Historic Places in 1983. All of the more than 100 pieces of furniture in the lodge was crafted from two myrtlewood logs 5 feet in diameter and 40 feet long.

The nearby town of Silverton is home to the Silverton Historical Museum, a 1908 home which offers more photographs and artifacts from the area's farming and logging history. Visit in July to catch the annual Al Faussett Days festival, commemorating Faussett's 1928 plunge over South Falls in a canvas canoe. Present-day Faussett family members converge at the falls along with hundreds of visitors who are treated to a newsreel of the actual event—and an "old fashioned pie social."

While many campgrounds are mere jumping-off points for nearby attractions, Silver Falls is one area that neatly encompasses all activities in its boundaries. Cabins are also available for rent, and there are several group-camping sites as well. Although the park does tend to get a little crowded because it's so popular—and long has been, even decades before the first land was deeded to the state for a park—it's also quite easy to lose the crowds because of its sheer size.

Despite the area's name, no one has struck it rich mining silver, gold, or any other ore here, but the park's natural wonders are a perfect example of our most precious commodities.

KEY INFORMATION

ADDRESS: Silver Falls Campground 20024 Silver Falls Highway SE Sublimity, OR 97385

OPERATED BY: Oregon State Parks

INFORMATION: (503) 873-8681, (800) 551-6949; www.oregon stateparks.org

OPEN: April–October

SITES: 100

EACH SITE: Picnic table, fire ring

ASSIGNMENT: First-come, first-served, or by reservation at (800) 452-5687 or www .reserveamerica .com ($6 fee)

REGISTRATION: At park entrance

FACILITIES: Flush toilets, hot showers

PARKING: At campsites and at park entrance

FEE: $12; $5 per additional vehicle

ELEVATION: 250 feet

RESTRICTIONS: *Pets:* On leash only (dogs are not allowed on the Trail of Ten Falls) *Fires:* In fire rings only *Alcohol:* At campsites only *Vehicles:* 1 per site *Other:* 14-day stay limit

MAP

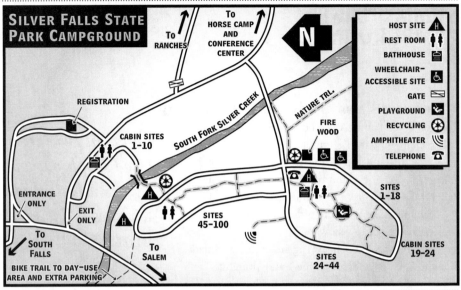

GETTING THERE

From Salem, drive east on OR 22 for 5 miles to OR 214. Turn left, and drive 15 miles to the park entrance.

GPS COORDINATES

UTM Zone (WGS84)   10T
Easting   0527488
Northing   4968990
Latitude   N 44.8738°
Longitude   W 122.652°

THE NAME'S A BIT MISLEADING, as there is no sense of having reached the top of something when you get to Summit Lake. But once you're here, you'll be on top of the world and so proud of yourself for having found this wonderfully simple yet delightful spot far from the Timothy Lake crowds.

Summit Lake is on the order of Rujada (see page 136)—a great place to visit when you don't have a lot of time and don't want a heavy agenda. Unlike Rujada, Summit Lake is underdeveloped and primitive, with mostly walk-in sites either anchored by the shoreline or on a slight inland incline with a lake view.

Access to Summit Lake is almost too easy, which is what makes the lack of crowds so surprising. It could be that the magnetic draw of Timothy Lake, with its eye-popping views of Mount Hood, is all it takes to divert impressionable campers. It also could be that those who value a sublime place like Summit Lake aren't about to share it with others. The most plausible theory of all is that most people are driving way too fast on the Oregon Skyline Road (a.k.a. Forest Service 42) to see the very small, dark-brown wooden sign engulfed in roadside foliage pointing the way to Summit Lake down FS 141.

Whatever the reasons, Summit Lake shows up on detailed topographic maps as the tiniest blue slash alongside the Skyline Road, and those of us who have discovered its charms hope the campground retains its rustic, untrammeled character.

Here's a simple lesson in how to enjoy Summit Lake: Drive the mile of decent gravel off the Skyline Road down FS 141, park the car in the group-parking area, take a short walk along one of the camp trails, pick the spot of your choice (you may not have as many choices on the weekend), and then unload the car. Total time from turning off Skyline Road: 20 minutes.

> *Summit Lake is small and simple but with generously sized walk-in sites—all with lake views.*

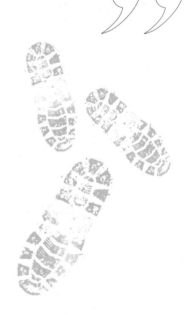

RATINGS

Beauty: ✰ ✰ ✰ ✰
Privacy: ✰ ✰ ✰ ✰
Spaciousness: ✰ ✰ ✰ ✰ ✰
Quiet: ✰ ✰ ✰ ✰ ✰
Security: ✰ ✰ ✰ ✰ ✰
Cleanliness: ✰ ✰ ✰ ✰ ✰
Insect control: ✰ ✰ ✰

ADDRESS: Summit Lake
Campground
c/o Zigzag Ranger
District
70220 East US 26.
Zigzag, OR 97049

OPERATED BY: Thousand Trails
for Mount Hood
National Forest

INFORMATION: (503) 622-3191

OPEN: Late May–
September

SITES: 5

EACH SITE: Picnic table, fire
grill

ASSIGNMENT: First come,
first served; no
reservations

REGISTRATION: Self-registration
on site

FACILITIES: Vault toilets,
piped water,
garbage service

PARKING: In parking area

FEE: $12

ELEVATION: 4,200 feet

RESTRICTIONS: *Pets:* On leash only
Fires: In fire pits
only
Alcohol: Permitted
Vehicles: 16-foot
RV size limit, no
hookups
Other: 14-day limit
on stay; nonmotor-
izeboats only on
lake

Summit Lake will appear on your left as you drive along FS 141, so enjoy the preview. Campsites 1 and 2 are the only drive-in sites, but I don't consider them the best sites because they have very little privacy and are opposite the parking area for the walk-in sites. I imagine it gets noisy and busy with engines starting, doors slamming (there should be a camp rule against this), and gear being transported.

Go for sites 4 and 5 if you can. These are the farthest from the parking area so toting a lot of stuff can be a bit of a drag, and you have to pass the other campsites getting there. (Keep to the trail; cutting through other campsites is a major camping faux pas.) Sites 4 and 5 offer the best vantage for enjoying lake views and those early morning sunrises. Site 3 isn't all bad, but it sits fairly near the parking area. Sites 7 and 8 sit back from the lake but are bounded on all sides by the trails that lead through the campground, perhaps an annoying element when children are chasing each other through the underbrush oblivious to your tent nearby. Site 6 sits alone up a small grade and has the best overview of the lake and the other campsites.

In general, the sites are spacious with a smattering of foliage in between to soften the views, but I would not describe the underbrush as lush or the campsites as shrouded. A tent positioned in the right way can do a lot to act as a curtain. What these sites lack in privacy, however, they make up for by being spaced well apart. Each has the basic amenities—picnic table and grill—and they share a modern vault toilet near the parking area. Garbage services are a notable plus.

The Oregon Skyline Road, which passes by Summit Lake, cuts a mid-elevation swath between the dense Mount Hood National Forest on its western flank and the rolling ridges of the Warm Springs Indian Reservation to the east. It ultimately meets up with FS 46, which continues northward as Clackamas River Road and becomes Breitenbush Road to the south before its junction with OR 22 at Detroit.

Recreational opportunities abound, with two scenic byways to explore, the "Wild and Scenic" Clackamas River to admire, trout-stocked lakes to tackle, and endless mountain ridges to wander. Bring a good map,

MAP

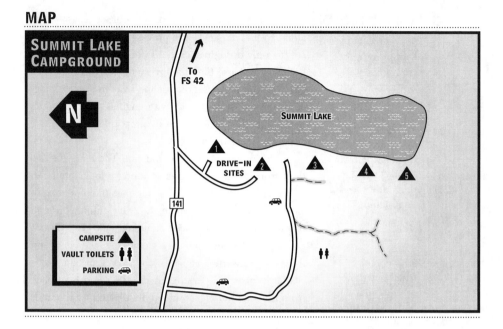

GETTING THERE

From the intersection of US 26 and OR 35 on the south side of Mount Hood (just past Government Camp), drive east on US 26 for 15 miles to FS 42 (also known as Skyline Road). Drive for 12 gravel miles to FS 141. The sign is nearly hidden by vegetation, so watch your mileage. Turn right onto FS 141 and follow it for about a mile. Summit Lake will be on your left.

GPS COORDINATES

UTM Zone (WGS84)	10T
Easting	0595312
Northing	4987328
Latitude	N 45.033°
Longitude	W 121.79°

a set of binoculars, a comfortable pair of boots, and however much time you can spare. You may not accomplish everything on this trip, but it's not too far to come back soon.

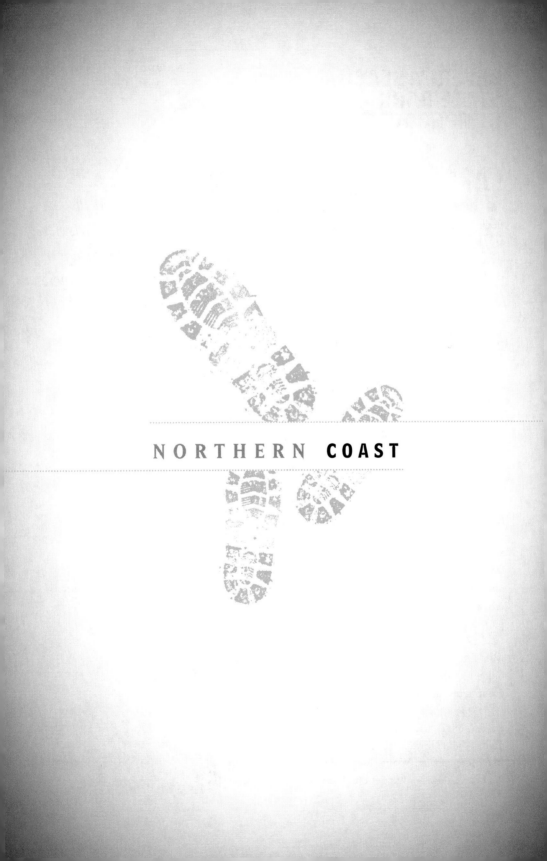

NORTHERN COAST

34

BEVERLY BEACH STATE PARK CAMPGROUND

WHILE YOU MAY THINK of the Pacific Coast as a summer destination, Oregon steps to the beat of a different drummer. Many people flock to the rugged Oregon coast to watch the winter storms and look out for whales. In fact, the prime whale-watching months are from late December to mid-March, when volunteers set up camp specifically to help you spot the spouts at prime locations along the coast.

Located seven miles north of Newport, Beverly Beach is a must-stay campground if you're in the area. While many of the surrounding campgrounds can get overloaded with RVs and consequently feel a little cramped, this campground manages to host everyone and still make you feel like you've gotten away from it all (and from your neighbor). The sites are spacious and wooded, and a nature trail winds its way through the campground, so you can get a little exercise to start off your day.

The most scenic part of the nature trail follows Spencer Creek, which borders the campground to the south. Access the trail near site C-7. After crossing Spencer Creek, the trail splits. Walking to the right takes you to the hiker/biker camp. Head left to walk along the creek. The trail follows the creek to a bridge crossing located near site G-16. If you like to bicycle, park roads are open to bikes (helmets required).

Divided into eight loops, the campground is large, with 128 tent sites—trailers of any kind are wisely forbidden in the tent-camping areas. There are also five group tent-camping areas.

One attraction of this campground is that you can walk to the beach from your tent site through a tunnel under the highway, allowing for front-row seats to watch the sun set. While there are some sites closer to the beach, they tend to get bombarded with visitors, so

> *You'll get all the creature comforts here, but you can also lose yourself in the spacious sites at this beachside campground.*

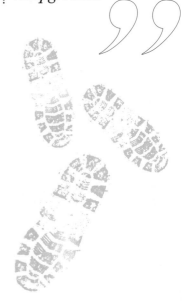

RATINGS

Beauty: ✿ ✿ ✿ ✿
Privacy: ✿ ✿ ✿
Spaciousness: ✿ ✿ ✿ ✿
Quiet: ✿ ✿
Security: ✿ ✿ ✿
Cleanliness: ✿ ✿ ✿
Insect Control: ✿ ✿ ✿

ADDRESS: Beverly Beach State Park 198 NW 123rd St. Newport, OR 97365

OPERATED BY: Oregon State Parks

INFORMATION: (541) 265-9278, (800) 452-5687; www.oregon stateparks.org

OPEN: Year-round

SITES: 128

EACH SITE: Picnic table, fire ring

ASSIGNMENT: First come, first served; or by reservation at (800) 452-5687 or www .reserveamerica .com ($6 fee)

REGISTRATION: At the campground entrance

FACILITIES: Flush toilets, hot showers

PARKING: At campsites only

FEE: Tent sites are $13 per night (October–April); $17 (May– September)

ELEVATION: Sea level

RESTRICTIONS: *Pets:* On leash only *Fires:* In fire rings only *Alcohol:* Permitted *Vehicles:* 1 per site; $5 per additional vehicle *Other:* 14-day stay limit

don't be fooled into thinking those are the best spots. Generally, the farther you are from the beach, the more likely you are to have some solitude. If you like to surf, the north beach is recommended. If you want to look for fossils, walk south along the beach.

With a general store nearby, firewood available at the campground, and a campground entrance station where staff will fill you in on the recreation hot spots—not to mention flush toilets and hot showers—Beverly Beach is a prime spot for tent-camping luxury with some elbow room.

Hiking is a popular activity here, with plenty of lighthouses (in particular, Yaquina Head lighthouse is just south of the campground) and viewpoints to explore right off famous US 101. Of course, simply driving is a sight-seeing exploration in itself, as the sweeping cliff-side views of waves crashing below will tempt you to get out of your car and take advantage of the viewpoints. Just north of Cape Foulweather, visit Depoe Bay and its remarkable spouting horn. When ocean waves surge into rocky tunnels along the shore, the spout erupts á la Old Faithful.

In addition, Newport is 7 miles south, so you can get a fix of coastal city charm at the historic waterfront (and sample some famous Moe's Clam Chowder). Established in 1882, Newport is a small town along the Yaquina bay waterfront. Newport also has charter rentals, if you want to get out on the water, and the Oregon Coast Aquarium is just a few miles away. In fact, there's so much to do in the surrounding area, it's a good thing Beverly Beach is open year-round, so you can pick your pleasure.

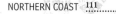

MAP

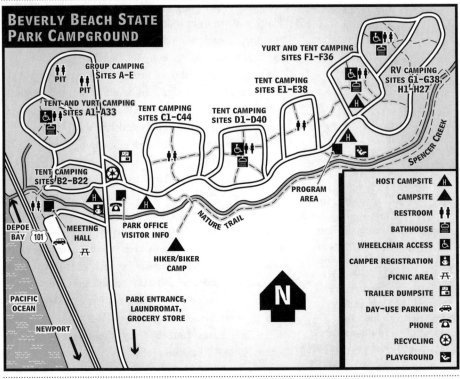

BEVERLY BEACH STATE PARK CAMPGROUND

GROUP CAMPING SITES A-E
PIT
PIT

TENT-AND YURT CAMPING SITES A1-A33

TENT CAMPING SITES C1-C44

TENT CAMPING SITES D1-D40

TENT CAMPING SITES E1-E38

TENT CAMPING SITES B2-B22

YURT AND TENT CAMPING SITES F1-F36

RV CAMPING SITES G1-G38, H1-H27

SPENCER CREEK

PROGRAM AREA

NATURE TRAIL

DEPOE BAY 101

MEETING HALL

PARK OFFICE VISITOR INFO

HIKER/BIKER CAMP

PACIFIC OCEAN

NEWPORT

PARK ENTRANCE, LAUNDROMAT, GROCERY STORE

N

HOST CAMPSITE	H
CAMPSITE	▲
RESTROOM	�[
BATHHOUSE	⌷
WHEELCHAIR ACCESS	♿
CAMPER REGISTRATION	🛈
PICNIC AREA	🛆
TRAILER DUMPSITE	⊡
DAY-USE PARKING	🚗
PHONE	☎
RECYCLING	♺
PLAYGROUND	🛝

GPS COORDINATES

UTM Zone (WGS84)	10T
Easting	0416257
Northing	4953102
Latitude	N 44.7264°
Longitude	W 124.0575°

GETTING THERE

From Newport, drive 7 miles north on US 101 to the park entrance on the right (east) side of the highway.

35
CAPE LOOKOUT STATE PARK CAMPGROUND

> *Superb views, wildlife refuges, and historic sites make Cape Lookout a popular destination for weekenders and summer vacationers from Oregon's metropolitan areas.*

THE FIRST OF THREE CAMPGROUNDS in what I like to refer to as the "cape-camping collection" is the lovely and linear Cape Lookout State Park, just south of Netarts on the Three Capes Scenic Drive (for the other two campgrounds, see pages 153 and 156). The route actually encompasses two more state parks with (as you may have guessed from the road's name) magnificent headlands—Cape Meares on the north and Cape Kiwanda on the south—but these are day-use facilities only.

Capes Lookout, Meares, and Kiwanda are the centerpiece of more than 2,500 acres of coastal rain forest, sheer cliffs, wide sandy beaches and dunes, narrow spits, rocky points and outcroppings, protected bays, and estuaries.

To accommodate the sizable numbers of seashore enthusiasts, the well-maintained and efficiently designed Cape Lookout State Park offers a whopping 173 tent sites, many of which are accessible all year. In addition, it offers a separate (and quieter) hiker-and-biker camp not far from the central camping grounds. Group camps are also available, as well as a meeting hall and four cabins. Despite the number of campsites, there is a spaciousness and openness about the place so that it feels—dare I say it?—uncrowded. That's not likely to be the case on any given summer day, but enjoy the feeling when you can. It's due in large part to the fact that when you have your back to the cape, the view is mainly of sand dunes, saltwater, and sky, a heady combination that encourages mindless meandering and musing. But if you insist on a mission, consider shell collecting, birdwatching, whalespotting (at the right times of year), and the like.

Geologically speaking, it may come as a surprise that the exquisite cape formations in this area and all along the Oregon Coast are the wind-, weather-, and

RATINGS

Beauty: ✿ ✿ ✿ ✿ ✿
Privacy: ✿ ✿ ✿ ✿
Spaciousness: ✿ ✿ ✿
Quiet: ✿ ✿ ✿ (summer)
✿ ✿ ✿ ✿ (winter)
Security: ✿ ✿ ✿ ✿
Cleanliness: ✿ ✿ ✿ ✿ ✿
Insect Control: ✿ ✿ ✿

wave-carved remains of ancient volcanoes. Geologists speculate that massive Cape Lookout, considered by many to be one of the most scenic capes in the Northwest, originally formed as an island off the coast when a huge lava flow cooled and congealed differently above and below sea level. You can observe the geologic layers from the base of this 700-foot promontory. The Cape Meares formation occurred similarly.

Cape Kiwanda, however, is essentially compressed sand made into rock and then shoved upward. Its sandstone composition would normally make Cape Kiwanda a fragile target of the pounding surf, but as if by a master plan, nature provided the lofty point with its own Haystack Rock. (The more famous one is farther north, off the coast of Cannon Beach.) This giant piece of basalt encumbers incoming waves so effectively that fishing boats can head directly into the subdued breakers. In honor of this phenomenon, Pacific City (south of Cape Kiwanda) holds the Pacific City Dory Derby each summer, showing off the seafaring talents of its famous fleet of flat-bottomed boats.

The Cape Meares cliffs are the nesting grounds for a wide variety of shorebirds that are protected, along with their forest-dwelling counterparts, by Cape Meares National Wildlife Refuge and Three Arch Rock National Wildlife Refuge in Oceanside. Between the two refuges, more than 150 species of birds are known to inhabit the shores and uplands. Cape Meares is also the site of the "Octopus Tree," a Sitka spruce gone wild, with an inordinate number of drooping branches. Historic Tillamook Light lighthouse on Cape Meares is the structural centerpiece of this park. You'll also have a decent chance of seeing elk on the Cape Meares Hiking Trail.

The average 90 inches of annual rainfall keep things fairly wet in winter and struggling to dry out in summer. If you dress appropriately, hiking the headlands and watching storms roll in can be an exhilarating winter adventure along this stretch of Oregon coast. The Cape Lookout Trail alone traces the headland for more than 2 miles and winds up at a clifftop 500 feet above the sea. There are a total of 8 miles of trails through old-growth forest in the park. Several trails offer interpretive signage noting indigenous foliage and

KEY INFORMATION

ADDRESS:	Cape Lookout State Park 13000 Whiskey Creek Road W Tillamook, OR 97141
OPERATED BY:	Oregon State Parks
INFORMATION:	(503) 842-4981, (800) 551-6949; www.oregon stateparks.org
OPEN:	Year-round
SITES:	173 tent; 38 full-hookup, 1 electric; group site and hiker/biker camp
EACH SITE:	Picnic table, fire pit and grill, piped water, shade trees
ASSIGNMENT:	First come, first served; or by reservation at (800) 452-5687 or www .recreation.gov
REGISTRATION:	On site
FACILITIES:	Flush toilets, hot water, showers; day-use area ($3 per vehicle) has picnic tables, grills, and beach access; limited disabled access
PARKING:	At campsites
FEE:	Tents $16, $12 winter; full hookups $20, $16 winter; deluxe cabins $66, $45 winter; yurts $27; hiker/biker sites $4 per person; $5 per additional vehicle
ELEVATION:	Sea level
RESTRICTIONS:	*Pets:* On leash only *Fires:* In fire pits *Alcohol:* Permitted *Vehicles:* No limit *Other:* 14-day limit

MAP

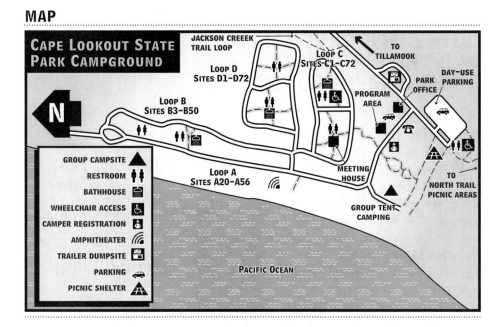

Cape Lookout State Park Campground

- GROUP CAMPSITE
- RESTROOM
- BATHHOUSE
- WHEELCHAIR ACCESS
- CAMPER REGISTRATION
- AMPHITHEATER
- TRAILER DUMPSITE
- PARKING
- PICNIC SHELTER

JACKSON CREEEK TRAIL LOOP

LOOP D SITES D1–D72

LOOP C SITES C1–C72

TO TILLAMOOK

DAY–USE PARKING

PROGRAM AREA

PARK OFFICE

LOOP B SITES B3–B50

LOOP A SITES A20–A56

MEETING HOUSE

GROUP TENT CAMPING

TO NORTH TRAIL PICNIC AREAS

PACIFIC OCEAN

GETTING THERE

To reach Cape Lookout from Tillamook, drive southwest on Netarts Highway, following signs for Cape Lookout State Park the entire way. The total distance from Tillamook is about 10 miles without any detours or side trips.

GPS COORDINATES

UTM Zone (WGS84) 10T
Easting 0424665
Northing 5024104
Latitude N 45.3664°
Longitude W 123.962°

salmon restoration efforts. Keep in mind that many of these trails are steep and slick in places. Safer and equally as interesting is the 5-mile stroll along Cape Lookout State Park's sand spit, between the ocean and Netarts Bay. You should also consider taking a trip from the upper trailhead down to South Beach.

In the bay's calm waters, you'll find conditions ideal for crabbing, either by boat or from the shore. Supplies can be found in town, and several places will cook your catch for you. Clamming and fishing are other options.

If you run out of things to do (which is unlikely) and want to play tourist, Tillamook is nearby. It has a history museum and tours of its renowned cheese factory. If you're wondering about those huge aluminum barns you can see from US 101 out in the middle of a pasture, that's the Tillamook Air Museu, which features more than 30 "War Birds" and actual pieces of the Hindenburg.

36

DOVRE, ELK BEND, AND THE NESTUCCA RIVER CAMPGROUNDS

NOT TOO FAR OUT THERE, but definitely "out there," a series of campgrounds on the Nestucca River are easily accessible via the official Nestucca Back Country Byway. You'll have the distinct feeling that you've stumbled upon someone's private party when you arrive at these campgrounds. They're that intimate—and largely unknown to the hordes that congregate along the coast.

Four Bureau of Land Mangement sites and one Forest Service facility comprise the Nestucca River chain of campgrounds; from east to west, they are Dovre, Fan Creek, Elk Bend, Alder Glen, and Rocky Bend. Collectively, they offer an extraordinary selection of 43 tent-camping sites spread across 12 miles of beautiful forested river frontage, so I decided to lump them all together. Take your pick or try them all.

The three campgrounds highlighted here are under the jurisdiction of the BLM's Tillamook Resource Area. True to BLM management style, the sites along the Nestucca are well-designed (albeit compact), primitive sites tucked along the banks of the river. They range in altitude from 700 feet at Rocky Bend up to 1,500 feet at Dovre.

Of the five, as far as tent camping goes, Elk Bend has the most going for it. It is walk-in only with five sites, and there is no fee. Rocky Bend has six sites and is also free, but it is not walk-in; the three other campgrounds have either 10 or 11 campsites and the fee is $10 per night and $5 for each additional vehicle. Elk Bend and Rocky Bend stay open all year long; the others operate between early April and the end of November.

All campgrounds have piped water except Rocky Bend. All but Elk Bend offer wheelchair accessibility at some sites. Picnic tables and fire pits are standard issue in each campsite. Dovre has one group shelter with its own fire pit. Alder Glen sports its own fishing pier. All garbage must be packed out of all sites.

> *Take your pick from this trio of BLM campgrounds that offer solitude, scenery and riverside settings.*

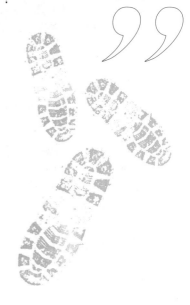

RATINGS

Beauty: ✩ ✩ ✩ ✩ ✩
Privacy: ✩ ✩ ✩
Spaciousness: ✩ ✩ ✩
Quiet: ✩ ✩ ✩ ✩
Security: ✩ ✩
Cleanliness: ✩ ✩ ✩ ✩ ✩
Insect Control: ✩ ✩

KEY INFORMATION

ADDRESS: Bureau of Land Management Tillamook Resource Area 4610 Third Street Tillamook, OR 97141

OPERATED BY: Bureau of Land Management

INFORMATION: (503) 815-1100

OPEN: April–November

SITES: 43 total

EACH SITE: Picnic table, fire grill

ASSIGNMENT: First come, first served; no reservations

REGISTRATION: Self-registration on site

FACILITIES: Vault toilets, solar-pumped water, group shelter with fire grill (Dovre has shelter)

PARKING: At campsites

FEE: $10; $5 per additional vehicle

ELEVATION: 700–1,500 feet

RESTRICTIONS: *Pets:* On leash only *Fires:* In fire pits only *Alcohol:* Permitted *Vehicles:* RVs up to 21 feet; no hookups *Other:* 14-day stay limit; only some sites are wheelchair accessible

Unless you're an avid angler, don't even think about vying for a spot along the Nestucca during the height of fall steelhead or spring and summer chinook runs. The river is known throughout the western hemisphere for its excellent runs of both species, as well as a year-round stocked supply of cutthroat trout.

If you are a paddler, be mindful that running the river at its peak (most likely when the fish are running as well) carries the risk of getting tangled in fishing lines. (Upper portions of the Nestucca River are non-navigable) Hopefully, there's room for everyone. The rains in winter can produce a good volume of water for boaters, but the river can also achieve flood stage quickly. Use common sense, and certainly don't boat alone in peak-flow periods.

The main attraction of the Nestucca Scenic Byway is the river itself and activities that relate to it. However, the coast and all its fascinations are not far away. Driving through the lowland meadows and farmlands on your way there, you may get sidetracked by the quaint villages that stay alive thanks to busy US 101 but retain a few artifacts from their pre-tourism heritage. Don't blink or you'll miss Blaine, where the Nestucca Byway takes a hard left to the west. Then comes Beaver at the byway's junction with US 101. Heading south, Hebo is home to the district office of the Siuslaw National Forest, a good place for maps and information. Cloverdale calls itself "Oregon's Best Kept Secret," and I guess most people who breeze through would agree.

Hiking options are not immediately apparent at the Nestucca campgrounds. The forest lands surrounding the Nestucca River are broken up into a mix of federal, state, and private stewardship. It's difficult to know whose territory you might be invading, so it is a good idea to check with either the Siuslaw National Forest, BLM, or Tillamook State Forest authorities. Recognizable hiking trails are not too far away on Mount Hebo, where you can walk through some very old second-growth forest or clamber along an even older pioneer road converted to trail. Although there's a trail to the summit of Mount Hebo for die-hard hikers, you can also drive up for expansive views of the Nestucca Valley and west to the Pacific.

MAP

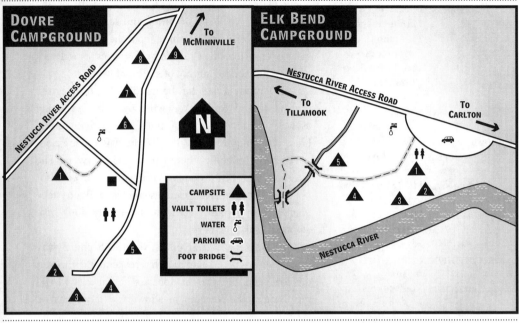

GETTING THERE

From SR 47 in Carlton (north of Mc-Minnville), turn west on Meadow Lake Road, which becomes Nestucca River Access Road (also known as the Nestucca Scenic Byway). Follow this 17 miles to the campground. There are numerous side roads that depart from the main road, so check road signs occasionally to make sure you're on the right track. From the coast, the Nestucca River Road is accessed off US 101 in Beaver on Blaine Road just north of Hebo. Once again, follow signs as the road takes many jogs and twists.

GPS COORDINATES

UTM Zone (WGS84) 10T
Easting 0457254
Northing 5014056
Latitude N 45.2787°
Longitude W 123.545°

37
SADDLE MOUNTAIN STATE PARK CAMPGROUND

If the summer crowds on the Oregon coast are more than you can handle but you don't want to forego scenic pleasures, consider Saddle Mountain State Park.

RATINGS

Beauty: ✿ ✿
Privacy: ✿ ✿ ✿
Spaciousness: ✿ ✿
Quiet: ✿ ✿
Security: ✿ ✿
Cleanliness: ✿ ✿ ✿ ✿
Insect Control: ✿ ✿ ✿ ✿

WANT TO ENJOY THE BEACH, see the mountains, and not get trampled by the crowds? Saddle Mountain is the answer.

Most people hurrying along US 26 between Portland and the ocean beaches in northwestern Oregon pass up this cool, green spot, either because they don't know about it or they have an unusual idea of "getting away from it all" in the overdeveloped, overpriced, and overrun resorts, motels, inns, rental cottages, and RV parks in seaside towns.

Don't get me wrong. I love the Oregon coast. If you want to pay the price, there are scads of wonderful places to stay—for a day, weekend, or week. And there are still plenty of areas that have been preserved in an undeveloped state to showcase the natural coastal beauty. But if your interest is tent camping in the purest sense, the Oregon coast may be a disappointment. You'll have to sacrifice ocean proximity for optimum peace and quiet by going farther inland to places such as Saddle Mountain State Park.

However, you have the best of both worlds at Saddle Mountain, because you'll be less than 15 miles from the nearest coastal attractions of Cannon Beach and Seaside, well away from the crowded US 101 corridor, and only a 2.6-mile hike from superb views from atop the park's namesake, the highest peak in northwestern Oregon. Not a bad combination, really.

Add to that a campground (albeit primitive) for tent campers only and nearly 3,000 acres (roughly 5 square miles) of second-growth forests, fragile meadows, and clear-running creeks. You'll share the terrain with a number of woodland critters (elk have been spotted in sizeable herds within the park) and a host of indigenous plantlife (more than 300 species have been identified), some that for reasons not altogether clear have chosen Saddle Mountain as their preferred habitat, growing only here and nowhere else in the Coast Range.

This latter feature will be of particular interest to the weekend botanist. Saddle Mountain was a haven for certain species of plant life during the Ice Age, and much of that flora evolved in ways peculiar to the Coast Range. Today, high on the flanks of this 3,283-foot peak, grow plants not found anywhere else. Patterson's bittercress is the most unique, found only on Saddle Mountain and nearby Onion Mountain. The best time to visit Saddle Mountain is early to mid-June, when the alpine wildflowers put on one of the most colorful shows in the region.

For the weekend mountaineer, Saddle Mountain Trail is a pleasantly surprising challenge, with a reward of unending views from the summit. Casual hikers will probably want to stop at the saddle just beyond the wildflower fields. The more adventurous and sure-footed in your party can continue on to the crest, but be forewarned that the path is steep and indistinct in places, making travel, as the park brochure says, "extremely treacherous" and not recommended for those who aren't in the best of shape.

Those who do make it to the top can feast on the views while enjoying a picnic lunch. To the south are Nehalem Bay and a sprinkle of small, characteristic coastal towns. Looking west, the Pacific Ocean paints a blue-green backdrop to the resort towns of Seaside and Cannon Beach, with Tillamook Head and Haystack Rock figuring prominently between them. Northward is historic Astoria where the Columbia River meets the Pacific. Fort Clatsop is the site of Lewis and Clark's winter camp in 1805 and 1806. Snowcapped Cascade Mountain peaks to the east add a finishing touch.

The weather is not always conducive to uninter-rupted vistas—or even a human presence—on the slopes of Saddle Mountain and can easily change for the worse between the time you leave your campsite and make the roundtrip hike of less than 7 miles. With an eleva-tion differential of more than 2,000 feet, the tempera-ture is often much warmer at the campground than at the summit, too, so keep that in mind as you pack. Ocean breezes can also have a chilling effect, even if the sun is bright. And in the most fierce conditions, the maritime Pacific climate has been known to dump upwards of 100 inches of rain annually, so be prepared for wet conditions anytime.

KEY INFORMATION

ADDRESS:	Saddle Mountain State Park P.O. Box 681 Cannon Beach, OR 97110
OPERATED BY:	Oregon State Parks
INFORMATION:	(503) 368-5943
OPEN:	April–November
SITES:	10
EACH SITE:	Picnic table, fire pit, piped water, shade trees
ASSIGNMENT:	First come, first served; no reservations
REGISTRATION:	Self-registration on site
FACILITIES:	Restrooms with toilets, sinks, running water; firewood
PARKING:	In campground
FEE:	$9; $5 per addi-tional vehicle
ELEVATION:	1,650 feet
RESTRICTIONS:	*Pets:* On leash only *Fires:* In fire pits only *Alcohol:* Permitted *Vehicles:* No RV or trailer accommodations; self-contained units may use parking lot *Other:* 14-day stay limit

MAP

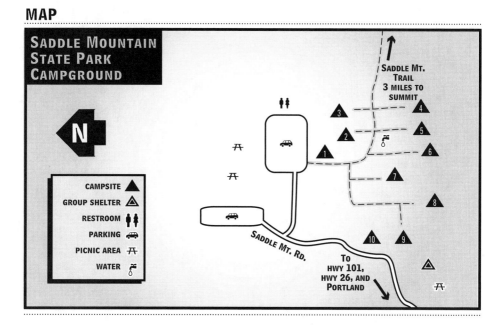

SADDLE MOUNTAIN STATE PARK CAMPGROUND

N

SADDLE MT. TRAIL 3 MILES TO SUMMIT

CAMPSITE ▲
GROUP SHELTER ⌂
RESTROOM ♀♂
PARKING 🚗
PICNIC AREA ⊼
WATER ⌐

SADDLE MT. RD.

TO HWY 101, HWY 26, AND PORTLAND

GETTING THERE

To reach Saddle Mountain State Park, turn north on Saddle Mountain Road off US 26 about 1.5 miles east of Necanicum Junction. Drive 7 miles to the campground. A picnic area, parking lot (self-contained RVs can park here), and trailhead are all located here as well.

GPS COORDINATES

UTM Zone (WGS84) 10T
Easting 0446536
Northing 5090157
Latitude N 45.9629°
Longitude W 123.69°

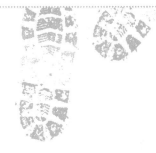

SOUTHERN **CASCADES**

38
FOURMILE LAKE CAMPGROUND

VIEWS OF A 9,500-FOOT SNOWCAPPED PEAK, spacious, lakefront tent sites wonderfully free of annoying mosquitoes (well, most of the year), a wilderness boundary practically at the backflap of your tent, trailheads to some of the wildest high-elevation territory in Oregon, a vast national wildlife refuge less than 20 miles away, regular security patrols, and the services of civilization within an hour's drive. It's hard to beat this glowing set of credentials, which is all part of the package when you stay at Fourmile Lake Campground in Fremont-Winema National Forest.

Although Fourmile's campsites are sizable enough to accommodate RVs, the general sense of the place is one of solitude and serenity. This is due, in part, to the proximity of Sky Lakes Wilderness, whose boundary is outlined by nearly three-fourths of the lake's shoreline.

Creating this squiggly crook in the wilderness's otherwise linear demarcation, Fourmile Lake is not within the protected boundaries, and motorized boat travel (with enforced speed limits) is acceptable. Any form of mechanized transportation within the wilderness territory is, however, strictly prohibited.

As always when hiking into wilderness backcountry, it is a good idea to carry a compass and a detailed USGS topographic map of the area. Forest Service maps are generally reliable but are often not updated frequently enough to reflect the most recent additions or changes in their vast network of roads. Try to get the most current information from a Forest Service representative. They're very friendly and helpful in Klamath Falls.

Hiking is required to enjoy this area properly, so carefully consider your options in either Sky Lakes Wilderness or Mountain Lakes Wilderness. Trails into Sky Lakes begin very near the campground. The one to the northwest passes diminutive Squaw Lake (where views

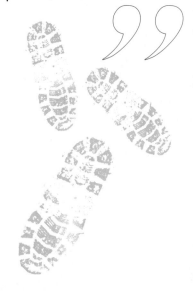

If you're campground shopping in the southern Oregon Cascades, it's hard to beat these fabulous views, lakefront sites, and wilderness trails.

RATINGS

Beauty: ✪ ✪ ✪ ✪
Privacy: ✪ ✪ ✪
Spaciousness: ✪ ✪ ✪ ✪ ✪
Quiet: ✪ ✪ ✪ ✪
Security: ✪ ✪ ✪ ✪
Cleanliness: ✪ ✪ ✪ ✪ ✪
Insect control: ✪ ✪ ✪ ✪

ADDRESS:	Fourmile Lake Campground c/o Klamath Ranger District 2819 Dahlia Street Klamath Falls, OR 97601
OPERATED BY:	Concessionaire for Fremont-Winema National Forest
INFORMATION:	(541) 885-3400
OPEN:	Late June–mid-October, weather permitting
SITES:	30
EACH SITE:	Picnic table, fire pit with grill, shade trees
ASSIGNMENT:	First come, first served; no reservations
REGISTRATION:	Self-registration on site
FACILITIES:	Vault toilets, central hand pumps for water, boat launch
PARKING:	At campsites
FEE:	$12; $6 per additional vehicle, $5 for day-use parking
ELEVATION:	5,800 feet
RESTRICTIONS:	*Pets:* On leash only *Fires:* In fire pits only *Alcohol:* Permitted *Vehicles:* Not allowed in wilderness area; nonmotorized boats only *Other:* 14-day stay limit

of Mount McLoughlin will make you stop and gawk) and soon thereafter connects with the Pacific Crest National Scenic Trail (about 2 miles from the campground). From there, you could hike south on the Pacific Crest Trail to its junction with the Mount McLoughlin Trail (a difficult but nontechnical climb). The summit is about 3 miles from this point. The trip from campground to peak would make for a rather rigorous 14-mile, round-trip day hike. The alternative is to hike the Mount McLoughlin Trail from its trailhead on FS 3650. An elevation gain of 4,000 feet doesn't make the trip any easier, but it is shorter (10 miles round-trip). Be sure to read the brochure that is provided at the trailhead. It covers some necessary precautions that can make the difference between delight and disaster on this fourth-highest Oregon Cascade volcano.

To experience the true essence of Sky Lakes Wilderness, I recommend driving to the Cold Springs trailhead on FS 3651. Saunter into the heart of this magnificent area with Imagination Peak as your inspiration. Beginning at an altitude of 5,800 feet, the trail climbs gently up and down without general elevation gain or loss.

In about 6 miles, you'll come to Heavenly Twin Lakes and the turnaround point if you're just out for the day. This is a good spot to see osprey that travel from nesting areas up to 8 miles away to fish in the hundreds of lakes scattered in this alpine basin. The trail wanders north past more peaks and lakes until it catches up with the Pacific Crest Trail as it works its way toward Crater Lake National Park.

South and east of Fourmile Lake is Mountain Lakes Wilderness, one of the oldest designated wilderness areas in Oregon and, for that matter, the entire country. The Forest Service included it in its Primitive Areas designations back in the 1930s, and it was incorporated under the 1964 Wilderness Act. Lesser known than the more popular destinations to the north but quite accessible from a trailhead at Sunset Campground, it may be the ticket for those seeking more solitary environs.

A challenging side trip—if you have the four-wheel rig to make it—is up Pelican Butte (also accessed from FS 3651). The Forest Service once manned a lookout station here, but the road is not maintained for

MAP

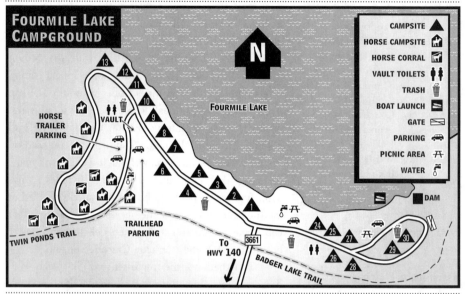

FOURMILE LAKE CAMPGROUND

FOURMILE LAKE

| CAMPSITE |
| HORSE CAMPSITE |
| HORSE CORRAL |
| VAULT TOILETS |
| TRASH |
| BOAT LAUNCH |
| GATE |
| PARKING |
| PICNIC AREA |
| WATER |

HORSE TRAILER PARKING

VAULT

TRAILHEAD PARKING

TWIN PONDS TRAIL

To HWY 140

3661

BADGER LAKE TRAIL

DAM

normal-clearance vehicles. Currently, Pelican Butte is officially designated as an 11,000-acre roadless area but a wilderness status is pending. No word on when this may be approved, but there is no doubt it would be a good thing for nature lovers.

Of course, hiking is not the only way to see this spectacular region. Rent a canoe down on Pelican Bay and follow Upper Klamath Canoe Trail through 6 miles of lake and marshland. An array of wildlife and water-fowl inhabit the 15,000 acres that comprise the Klamath National Wildlife Refuge

GETTING THERE

Take SR 140 (Lake of the Woods Highway) northwest out of Klamath Falls 38 miles, then turn right onto FS 3661, and head north 5.5 miles to the campground. From Medford, head east on SR 140 for 40 miles. From this direction, you will turn left onto FS 3661.

GPS COORDINATES

UTM Zone (WGS84)	10T
Easting	0561668
Northing	4700702
Latitude	N 42.4562°
Longitude	W 122.25°

39
HEAD OF THE RIVER CAMPGROUND

A great little out-of-the-way place where you'll run into more wildlife than people.

WE WERE SITTING IN A COFFEE SHOP in Klamath Falls, hard on the campground research trail. Besides the aroma of fresh-ground French roast opening up my drowsy, sleep-stagnant eyes, there was the unmistakable scent of a soon-to-be-discovered campground. You know, one of the campgrounds that the locals are afraid to tell anyone about—either because they fear the Forest Service will get wind of it and "undevelop" it to death or some sly, yuppie outdoor writer (hey, not me!) will want to tell the whole world about it.

As it turns out, my hunch was right. How do I get so lucky? You learn to recognize the signals quickly.

"Say, you wouldn't happen to know of any great little out-of-the-way camping spots around here, would you?" I asked innocently, with my nose stuck in a steaming mug.

The place wasn't very crowded, so it was obvious to the fellow behind the counter that the question was meant for him. He looked up with the tiniest twist of a smile, cocked his head to the side in exaggerated contemplation, pursed his lips, and said, "What do you mean by 'out-of-the-way?'"

He then told me about this dandy little spot known as Head of the River Campground. Lo and behold, I had actually seen it listed on campground lists—I guess I wasn't the first to play that game with the Klamath coffee connoisseur. They must have some arrangement with the Forest Service.

There isn't much to lure campers out to this tableland of ponderosa pine, lodgepole pine, and other conifers except a bit of excellent trout fishing in the Williamson River and a crazy contingent of Forest Service roads wandering in and around the numerous buttes and flats. The Forest Service would like to encourage more recreational use of these roads, which

RATINGS

Beauty: ✪ ✪ ✪ ✪
Privacy: ✪ ✪
Spaciousness: ✪ ✪ ✪ ✪
Quiet: ✪ ✪ ✪ ✪
Security: ✪
Cleanliness: ✪ ✪ ✪
Insect control: ✪ ✪ ✪

are primarily used by loggers. Problem is, they're too busy attending to the demands of campers in the overrun areas and don't have the budget to promote less-trammeled spots. When I talked with employees at both Chiloquin and Klamath Ranger Stations (Head of the River is located in the Chiloquin District but Klamath purports to manage it), they were polite and helpful from start to finish but scratched their heads at the notion that anyone would consider Head of the River and the surrounding terrain a place to seek out. But intrepid campers may be pleasantly surprised.

This area is relatively dry year-round, and the only substantial precipitation comes in the form of snow at higher elevations. However, enough groundwater seeps to the surface from natural springs (this is precisely the case with the headwaters of the Williamson) that wildflowers, such as fireweed, foxglove, lupine, and dandelion, define the banks of tiny, short-lived creeks every spring.

You'll most likely encounter more wildlife than fellow campers out here. More than 230 species of birds and 80 varieties of mammals inhabit the region. In the summer months, watch out for rattlesnakes and bring your mosquito repellent. Carry your own drinking water to Head of the River or be prepared to treat what you take from the river.

Rather than backtracking along the route you take to reach this pristine spot, consider a loop trip by continuing north on Williamson River Road, which becomes Silver Lake Road just above the expansive Klamath Marsh. You can get a close-up views of Klamath National Wildlife Refuge because Silver Lake Road cuts a diagonal across the refuge's midsection to a juncture with US 97 at Chinchalo. This could easily be one of the least-traveled byways you'll find in this book.

All in all, this is a remote area that begs to be appreciated simply for . . . well, its simplicity. The campground is as primitive as they come, with only five sites, no piped water, and no fee. For more specifics on the area, check either with the Chiloquin or Klamath Ranger District.

KEY INFORMATION

ADDRESS: Head of the River Campground c/o Chiloquin Ranger District 38500 OR 97 Chiloquin, OR 97624

OPERATED BY: Fremont-Winema National Forests, Klamath Ranger District

INFORMATION: (541) 783-4001

OPEN: May–October, weather permitting

SITES: 5

EACH SITE: Picnic table, shade trees

ASSIGNMENT: First come, first served; no reservations

REGISTRATION: Not necessary

FACILITIES: Wheelchair-accessible vault toilets, firewood, no potable water

PARKING: At campsites

FEE: No fee

ELEVATION: 4,500 feet

RESTRICTIONS: *Pets:* On leash only *Fires:* In fire pits only *Alcohol:* Permitted *Vehicles:* 30-foot RV size limit

MAP

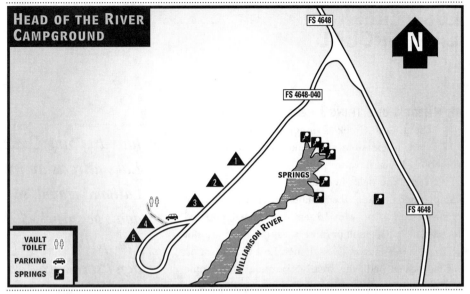

GETTING THERE

Take Sprague River Highway (OR 858) northeast out of Chiloquin. Take a left onto Williamson River Highway just beyond the 5-mile point. Follow this road 27 miles to the access road, FS 4648. Take a left; the campground is 1 mile on the left. Signs for the campground begin at the turn for FS 4648.

GPS COORDINATES

UTM Zone (WGS84)   10T
Easting   0628698
Northing   4733930
Latitude   N 42.7471°
Longitude   W 121.4275°

40
LOST CREEK CAMPGROUND

THERE'S ONE THING I NEED TO SAY right away about Lost Creek Campground: Get there as early as possible and stake your claim. Bribe somebody if you have to.

Here's the deal. Lost Creek is only one of two campgrounds inside the boundary of Crater Lake National Park. And with 16 tent-only sites—compared to Mazama's 213 multipurpose sites—the odds are not in a latecomer's favor. Even though Lost Creek is a bit off the beaten path, the area is swarming with people looking for overnight accommodations—roughly half a million visitors per year at last count. Many of them come from around the world. As acknowledgment of this, the park service offers trip-planning information in German, Spanish, and French on its Web site. I even encountered two German bicyclists who flew to Montana and were pedaling to Los Angeles via Crater Lake. I hope they made it. Nice to have so many cultures converging in such an unspoiled spot, actually. Natural beauty may make the best ambassador.

Oregon's only national park, which turned 100 years old in 2002, retains the stupendous natural wonders that garnered its protection in 1902. Park staff today feel that William Steel, the singular driving force behind the park's creation then, would be impressed with how little Crater Lake has changed in the course of a century. Besides the paving of formerly dirt roads, the only evident change is at Crater Lake Lodge, which underwent a multimillion-dollar remodeling in the early 1990s.

If this is your first trip to Crater Lake National Park, be prepared. Your jaw will drop when you take your first peek over the rim of this massive caldera. Everyone has an opinion on the best spot for your first good gawk but, frankly, that's just splitting hairs. The deepest lake in the United States, the second deepest in North America, and one of the 10 deepest in the world,

> *Jaw-dropping Crater Lake attracts an international crowd, so don't be surprised if your fellow campers don't speak English.*

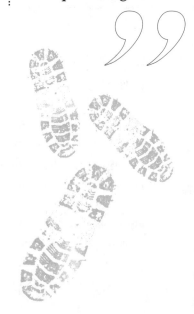

RATINGS

Beauty: ✰ ✰ ✰ ✰
Privacy: ✰ ✰ ✰ ✰ ✰
Spaciousness: ✰ ✰ ✰ ✰ ✰
Quiet: ✰ ✰ ✰ ✰ ✰
Security: ✰ ✰ ✰
Cleanliness: ✰ ✰ ✰ ✰
Insect control: ✰ ✰ ✰

KEY INFORMATION

ADDRESS: Lost Creek
Campground
Crater Lake
National Park
P.O. Box 7
Crater Lake, OR
97604

OPERATED BY: National Park
Service

INFORMATION: (541) 594-3100

OPEN: Early July–early
October, depend-
ing on snow level

SITES: 16

EACH SITE: Picnic table, fire
grill

ASSIGNMENT: First come,
first served; no
reservations

REGISTRATION: Self-registration
on site

FACILITIES: Flush toilets,
piped water

PARKING: At campsites

FEE: $10

ELEVATION: 6,000 feet

RESTRICTIONS: *Pets:* On leash only
Fires: In fire pits
only
Alcohol: At camp-
sites only
Vehicles: Motor-
bikes allowed; no
accommodations
for RVs

Crater Lake is the result of the cataclysmic eruption of Mount Mazama some 7,700 years ago. It once was a stratovolcano similar to Mount Hood and Mount Shasta and stood roughly a mile higher than the current lake level before it collapsed. There are several excellent publications about Crater Lake, Mount Mazama, and the park at the park's two visitor centers. I found it helpful to have these along as I toured the area. It's the kind of place where a little knowledge can make the trip immensely more pleasurable.

Rim Drive circumnavigates the perimeter of the 6-mile-wide lake for a total distance of 33.4 miles. There are numerous viewpoints along the way that will slow your driving time, but figure roughly two hours to complete the loop. In the winter, Rim Drive is open only between park headquarters and Rim Village, accessed by way of SR 62 from either the west or south. In all seasons, Rim Drive is open to bicycles, but there is no shoulder—so be careful!

Recreational activities in the 183,277 acres of Crater Lake National Park border on exhaustive, but the wanderer in you may want to simply observe on foot the diverse plant and animal life native to this part of Oregon. There are more than 140 miles of hiking trails (including a section of the Pacific Crest National Scenic Trail), and with so many of the park's visitors limiting their activity to areas closest to the crater's rim and park services, it is relatively easy to find solitude on a trail. Some trails reach elevations close to 9,000 feet and can take their toll on unconditioned legs and the unacclimatized cardiovascular system. Remember to carry water and take frequent rest stops to adjust to the altitude—and the incredibly fresh air.

For the geologist in you, there are destinations such as The Pinnacles (further down the road from Lost Creek Camp) and similarly weird formations on the Godfrey Glen Trail. The Pumice Desert is on the north side of the park, and Wizard Island, the small, symmetrical volcanic cone protruding from the lake, is accessible by boat from Cleetwood Cove. It's a steep, 720-foot drop on a trail just over a mile long to hike to the cove. The way down may seem manageable enough, but after several hours of hiking on Wizard Island, that

MAP

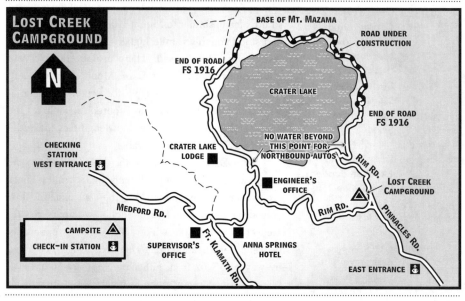

LOST CREEK CAMPGROUND

N

BASE OF MT. MAZAMA

ROAD UNDER CONSTRUCTION

END OF ROAD FS 1916

CRATER LAKE

END OF ROAD FS 1916

CHECKING STATION WEST ENTRANCE

CRATER LAKE LODGE

NO WATER BEYOND THIS POINT FOR NORTHBOUND AUTOS

RIM RD.

LOST CREEK CAMPGROUND

ENGINEER'S OFFICE

MEDFORD RD.

RIM RD.

PINNACLES RD.

CAMPSITE

CHECK-IN STATION

SUPERVISOR'S OFFICE

FT. KLAMATH RD.

ANNA SPRINGS HOTEL

EAST ENTRANCE

last mile back up may be the most memorable. Leave enough time to make the ascent in daylight.

Winter at Crater Lake is the dominant season, starting as early as October and lasting well into what is early summer in most places. Annual snowfall averages around 500 inches, which means endless winter-recreation opportunities if you're prepared. The park offers marked (but not groomed) cross-country skiing trails and snowmobile options. Most services in the park close in winter, but the cafe and gift shop at Rim Village stay open daily. Check the park's Web site for the most current conditions when considering a winter escape.

GETTING THERE

From Medford, follow SR 62 east 77 miles and turn left at the Annie Springs Entrance. Continue past Mazama Campground 4 miles, and turn right. Turn right just before the Phantom Ship Overlook toward The Pinnacles. Lost Creek Campground is adjacent to tiny Lost Creek several miles down this road.

GPS COORDINATES

UTM Zone (WGS84) 10T
Easting 0578564
Northing 4747905
Latitude N 42.8797°
Longitude W 122.038°

> *This is a good place to set up camp and explore the beautiful and often-overlooked Upper Rogue River area. Be sure to take a map!*

OFTEN OVERLOOKED BY TRAVELERS scurrying between the heavily promoted majesty of Crater Lake and the famed, lower "Wild and Scenic" Rogue River, the Upper Rogue River area offers its own style of spectacular scenery and wilderness treasures that should satisfy the desires of most outdoor adventurers.

If you're set on experiencing the beauty of the Rogue by boat, however, you'll be disappointed to discover that this section of the river is off limits to kayaks and canoes. Head on down to Grants Pass or the town of Rogue River, and they'll take care of you there.

Here, in Upper Rogue territory, the river plummets out of its source in Crater Lake National Park at a rate of as much as 48 feet per mile. Take a look down from precipitous heights along SR 62 north of Natural Bridge Campground for perhaps the clearest indication of why this portion of the river is so unrunnable. The flash of silver far below is the Rogue hurling itself seaward through the deep, narrow fissure known as the Rogue River Gorge.

Natural Bridge Campground is so named for the unique geological feature adjacent to it. In this location, the Upper Rogue disappears from sight and runs through an underground channel for 200 feet. The campground sits virtually atop the channel, with water flowing beneath it. A 2-mile interpretive loop trail explains the phenomenon.

Natural Bridge is one of several campgrounds in the vicinity located on the banks of the Rogue or on small creeks that feed it. Given its proximity to Crater Lake, this area can be quite busy in the summertime, but the larger, more developed campsites tend to fill up first. The lack of piped water or hookups at Natural Bridge discourages those who are not prepared for primitive conditions. The surrounding Rogue River

RATINGS

Beauty: ✪ ✪ ✪ ✪ ✪
Privacy: ✪ ✪ ✪ ✪ ✪
Spaciousness: ✪ ✪ ✪
Quiet: ✪ ✪ ✪ ✪
Security: ✪ ✪ ✪ ✪
Cleanliness: ✪ ✪ ✪ ✪ ✪
Insect control: ✪ ✪ ✪ ✪

National Forest is characterized by dense forests of Douglas fir and sugar pine, which soften the contours of the high plateau upon which they grow. More than 450 miles of trail within the national forest lead to remote high-country lakes, ridgetop vistas, and the secluded Rogue-Umpqua Divide Wilderness. Some of the routes connect with trails into the adjoining Umpqua National Forest.

Numerous day hikes and extended backpacking trips reveal not only the natural splendor of this undisturbed country but also the diverse wildlife and plant species that thrive in the moderate climate. The most famous inhabitant of Upper Rogue country is the northern spotted owl, which shares this lush expanse with an astonishing assortment of nocturnal creatures.

Except at the highest altitudes, which receive sizable measures of snow in the winter and stay cool year-round, the area enjoys warm and dry summers, with most of the 20 to 40 inches of annual precipitation occurring between October and May.

This rugged land is full of thick vegetation. Getting lost is easy. Make sure you have a good topographic or Forest Service map with you when you head out for lonely and distant spots. Booklets of maps and trail guides are available at the Rogue River National Forest headquarters in Medford or at the district office in Prospect.

If you are looking for an ambitious overland trek, take the Upper Rogue River Trail, which follows the river along its banks for 48 miles until it intersects with the Pacific Crest Trail in Crater Lake National Park. Starting in Prospect, the Upper Rogue Trail does not seem to attract as much print attention as its lower counterpart, known officially as the Rogue River National Recreation Trail. There's very little mention of the upper trail in regional guidebooks, so check in at the ranger station in Prospect, which is the best source for all outdoor recreation options in the area.

You can explore the trail in sections (who's got time for 48 miles all in one trip, anyway)? If you do have the time (and two cars or some kind of shuttle option), tackle the entire stretch and make daily destinations of the campgrounds sprinkled along the way,

KEY INFORMATION

ADDRESS:	Natural Bridge Campground c/o High Cascades Ranger District 47201 Crater Lake Highway Prospect, OR 97536
OPERATED BY:	Rogue River National Forest
INFORMATION:	(541) 560-3409
OPEN:	Late May until snow forces closure (typically in early November)
SITES:	17
EACH SITE:	Picnic table, fire pit with grill, shade trees
ASSIGNMENT:	First come, first served; no reservation
REGISTRATION:	Not necessary
FACILITIES:	Vault toilets, no piped water
PARKING:	At campsites
FEE:	$6, $3 per additional vehicle
ELEVATION:	2,900 feet
RESTRICTIONS:	*Pets:* On leash only *Fires:* In fire pits only *Alcohol:* Permitted *Vehicles:* 22-foot RV size limit

MAP

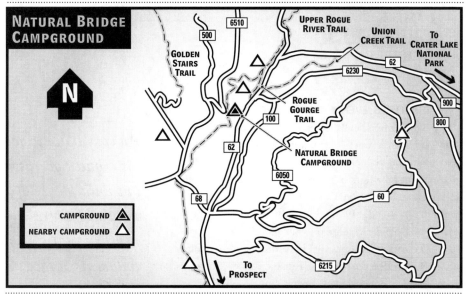

NATURAL BRIDGE CAMPGROUND

CAMPGROUND △
NEARBY CAMPGROUND △

GETTING THERE

Travel northeast on SR 62 (Crater Lake Highway) about 32 miles from Medford. From the Prospect turnoff, continue north on SR 62 another 11 miles or so to FS 300. Turn left, and the campground is 1 mile in. From Crater Lake, take SR 62 west if you are leaving the park from the south. If you exit from the north side, follow SR 138 to its intersection with SR 230. Head west and eventually south on SR 230 until it becomes SR 62. Turn right onto FS 300 about 3 miles from this point.

Natural Bridge included. This would be a fine way to spend a week getting intimately acquainted with the best of Upper Rogue country. Other options include shorter trails within a couple miles of the campground: The Natrual Bridge Interpretive Trail (0.3 miles) along the river often showcases beaver ponds; the Rogue Gorge Interpretive Trail (0.5 miles) also includes fascinating "pothole" formations in the rock, caused by the continuous spinning of small rocks in the water; and the Union Creek Trail (4.4 miles) follows the creek through a flower-filled old-growth Douglas fir forest to Union Falls.

GPS COORDINATES

UTM Zone (WGS84) 10T
Easting   0543686
Northing   4748561
Latitude   N 42.8884°
Longitude   W 122.465°

SOMETIMES EVEN A TENT-CAMPING guidebook like this one needs to recognize that every outing can't be a week-long planning and preparation extravaganza. Sometimes you just want a spot that doesn't require a tank of gas but still offers a rewarding forest experience. If you've only got a night to spare, welcome to Rujada. If you want to make it seem like a longer trip, head out there on your bicycle.

There is nothing particularly dramatic or exotic about Rujada. Except its name. Rujada, Rujada, Rujada. Don't have a clue what it means, but it rolls off the tongue in an alluring way. As you drive down the lane and cross the bridge over Layng Creek, you'll say, "Hey, what a great little campground. Why haven't we been here before?"

A mere 22 miles east of Cottage Grove up the Row River Road (which turns into FS 17), Rujada sits alone in creekside luxury at the base of Rose Hill. Rujada is located in the upper reaches of the Umpqua National Forest, a sprawling one million acres on the western slopes of the Cascades. The forest is characterized by the striking contrasts between cascading waterfalls, whitewater-river canyons, mountaintop vistas, and the ever-present green, green, green of ancient forests with shaggy coats of moss and lichen.

Rujada Campground is a microcosm of the Umpqua's ecosystems, with the clear and refreshing waters of Layng Creek at its feet, an expansive understory of ferns skirting its boundaries, stands of second-growth Douglas fir scattered throughout, and three dramatic waterfalls a short distance up FS 17: Moon Falls, Spirit Falls, and Pinard Falls.

The campground is laid out in classic, circular fashion as was the trend when campgrounds (including this one) were first developed by the Civilian Conservation Corps back in the 1930s. Evidence of its early

> *An easy place to reach for a quick overnight but with plenty of natural features nearby to satisfy your wilderness urges.*

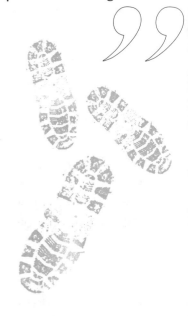

RATINGS

Beauty: ✿ ✿ ✿
Privacy: ✿ ✿ ✿ ✿ ✿
Spaciousness: ✿ ✿ ✿ ✿ ✿
Quiet: ✿ ✿ ✿ ✿
Security: ✿ ✿ ✿ ✿ ✿
Cleanliness: ✿ ✿ ✿ ✿ ✿
Insect Control: ✿ ✿ ✿

ADDRESS:	c/o Cottage Grove Ranger District 78405 Cedar Park Road Cottage Grove, OR 97427
OPERATED BY:	Umpqua National Forest
INFORMATION:	(541) 767-5000
OPEN:	Late May–September
SITES:	15
EACH SITE:	Picnic table, fire grill, shade trees
ASSIGNMENT:	First come, first served; no reservations
REGISTRATION:	Self-registration on site
FACILITIES:	Flush and vault toilets, piped water, garbage service, large day-use picnic areas surrounding an open grassy field for baseball or horseshoes, play equipment, swimming, camp host in high season
PARKING:	At campsites
FEE:	$8; $3 per additional vehicle
ELEVATION:	1,200 feet
RESTRICTIONS:	*Pets:* On leash only *Fires:* In fire pits only *Alcohol:* Permitted *Vehicles:* 22-foot RV size limit, no hookups *Other:* 14-day stay limit

origins is displayed at the historic register booth in the picnic area.

Most of Rujada's 15 sites are tucked deep into vegetated pockets, affording the ultimate in privacy. Site 4 is the closest in proximity to a delightfully private swimming hole on Layng Creek that attracts day users as well as campers. Knowledge of this particular swimming hole must rely heavily on word-of-mouth, because if the camp host hadn't told me about it, I doubt if I would have found it on my own (there's nothing at the campground advertising it, and dense underbrush keeps it hidden). Each campsite has plenty of space for a large tent and is appointed with a standard but sturdy wooden picnic table with the well-worn look of camping days gone by. The fire pits are concrete rings with grates.

Rujada is not the kind of campground that invigorates the soul to robust activity. Rather, it's a place of relaxation and serenity with perhaps a smattering of youthful vigor in the adjoining playing field with new playground equipment for small children as well as overhead bars for adult use (although I'm not quite sure what level of demand there is for its use). The first choice of activity for overworked adults in the immediate vicinity is hiking the Swordfern Trail, an easy walk just over a mile that follows Layng Creek partway, overtakes an old abandoned logging road, and completes its loop near the picnic area. If you're inclined to do more than this, the three waterfalls farther up FS 17 are must-sees and require little effort to reach their ultimate rewards. Catch Spirit Falls in early afternoon for the best photographic light, as it stays shrouded in shadows most of the day. Moon Falls is best viewed during periods of late spring or early summer runoff when the 125-foot plummet is at full tilt.

If this isn't enough to fill up your weekend, a drive up to Fairview Lookout and Musick Guard Station offers superb views and a taste of history. On the clearest of days, both Mount Hood to the north and Mount Shasta in California can be seen. The guardstation has been placed on the National Historic Register and the lookout (rebuilt in 1972) has served as a radar receptor in the past and is still used as a fire lookout during the peak of fire season (August and September). Both the

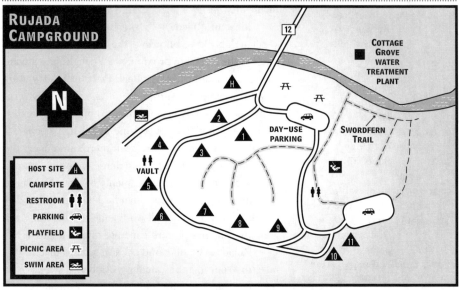

GETTING THERE

From Cottage Grove, take Row River Road east 19 miles to FS 17. Stay to the left and drive 2 miles to the campground entrance on the right. Cross Layng Creek and you're there.

cabin and lookout tower are available to rent. Pick up brochures for both facilities at the Cottage Grove Ranger District office.

If you have any time after these excursions, you may want to take the high-road route up and over Patterson Mountain that drops down into the Oakridge area. FS 17 switches to FS 5840 as it passes from Umpqua to Willamette National Forest, but I found my way to and from the Oakridge side with no problem. It's a little known back country drive that you can easily fit into a loose itinerary, and which may inspire you to return for another weekend.

GPS COORDINATES

UTM Zone (WGS84)	10T
Easting	0520706
Northing	4839330
Latitude	N 43.7067°
Longitude	W 122.743°

43
SACANDAGA CAMPGROUND

> *Waldo Lake, Diamond Peak, and the Willamette River are all within easy reach of Sacandaga.*

THE AREA SURROUNDING OAKRIDGE and Westfir is a forest playground for the outdoor-oriented masses of the Eugene-Springfield area. It is also becoming quite well-known (thanks in part to self-promotion) as a mountain-biking destination in the world beyond Oregon, but don't expect a hip, lively scene like that of other burgeoning Meccas for outdoor enthusiasts. It's still pretty quaint—which is not necessarily a bad thing! The number of churches outweighs the tavern listings on the Visitor's Map, if that tells you anything. I didn't spend too much time in town, but saw the standard assortment of modest local cafes and few fast-food eateries. I found good coffee (by Pacific Northwest standards) and pastries at The Trailhead Coffeehouse.

Oakridge is also a jumping-off point to High Cascades wonders in the southern Willamette National Forest, including Waldo Lake—one of the purest lakes in the world—and majestic Diamond Peak. Sacandaga Campground is close enough to town for conveniences but far enough away to be serene. It's safely away from the sometimes rowdy campers along nearby Hills Creek Reservoir and is definitely less overrun than supremely popular Waldo Lake, yet it's within day-tour driving distance of the High Cascades. At Sacandaga, the Middle Fork Willamette cuts through a narrow canyon that is seemingly far below but still emits up through the dense forest of Douglas fir, cedar, and hemlock one of the most pleasant campground sounds—the soothing constancy of a rushing river. A steep trail leads down to the river; walk cautiously in wet conditions, as it is easy to lose your footing.

At the campground, you'll find beautifully spacious campsites beneath a deep-forest canopy interspersed with dogwood trees. In my estimation, campsites 4, 6, and 8 are the best. Each sits on the edge of

RATINGS

Beauty: ✿ ✿ ✿ ✿ ✿
Privacy: ✿ ✿ ✿ ✿
Spaciousness: ✿ ✿ ✿ ✿ ✿
Quiet: ✿ ✿ ✿ ✿ ✿
Security: ✿ ✿ ✿ ✿
Cleanliness: ✿ ✿ ✿ ✿ ✿
Cleanliness: ✿ ✿ ✿

the bluff high above the river, the best vantage point for views and the sounds of the river right out of your tent door. Back in to your campsite, unload in relative privacy, and except for the occasional trip to the water faucet or the vault toilet, you can choose to have very little contact with other campers. Chances are these sites will be available, as the Forest Service rates this campground as seeing "low" usage, but you really can't go wrong anywhere within the camp if you don't get one of the prime spots.

Great driving tours are within easy reach of Sacandaga Campground, but one of the best tours can be enjoyed via foot, pedal, or hoof power right from the campground. The 27-mile-long Middle Fork Trail meanders through old-growth stands and meadows up and around the river, ending at the headwaters of its eponymous creek at Timpanogas Lake (see profile on page 145). The trail is open to hikers, horses, and mountain bikers; the lower part of the trail is considered a good introduction to serious mountain biking, with enough roots, rocks, and short climbs to challenge (but not discourage) a beginner. It also makes a great hike that even the youngest member of your party can enjoy. Sacandaga sits a little less than halfway along the trail, so you can choose routes in either direction.

Sections of the Middle Fork Trail follow the old Oregon Central Military Wagon Road, originally built in 1864 to bring cattle from the Willamette Valley over Emigrant Pass to the southern and eastern portions of the state. (It was eventually replaced by what is now OR 58 over Willamette Pass). The campground lies along the Diamond Drive Tour, which also follows part of the Military Wagon Road. The newly-designated route stretches south from Oakridge to SR 138 along the Rogue-Umpqua Scenic Byway, and provides excellent views of Diamond Peak, Mount Thielsen, and Sawtooth Mountain. Diamond Drive also connects on its north end to FS 19, also known as Aufderheide Scenic Byway. (The Auferheide is also part of the southern leg of the West Cascade Scenic Byway.) The Aufderheide tour starts near the longest covered bridge in Oregon, located in Westfir, and climbs along the rugged North Fork of the Middle Fork of the Willamette River, to the

KEY INFORMATION

ADDRESS: Sacandaga Campground c/o Middle Fork Ranger District 46375 OR 58 Westfir, OR 97492

OPERATED BY: Willamette National Forest

INFORMATION: (541) 782-2283

OPEN: June–October

SITES: 17

EACH SITE: Picnic table, fire pit

ASSIGNMENT: First-come, first-served; no reservations

REGISTRATION: Self-registration on site

FACILITIES: Vault toilets, piped water, garbage service

PARKING: At campsites

FEE: $8; $4 per additional vehicle

ELEVATION: 2,400 feet

RESTRICTIONS: *Pets:* On leash only *Fires:* In fire pits only *Alcohol:* Permitted *Vehicles:* 24-foot trailer size limit

MAP

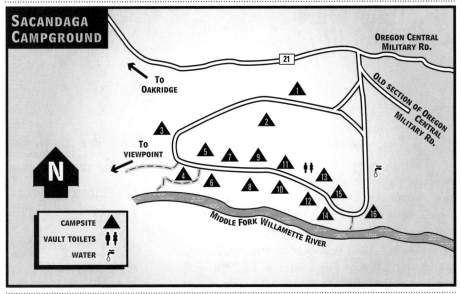

SACANDAGA CAMPGROUND

OREGON CENTRAL MILITARY RD.

21

To OAKRIDGE

OLD SECTION OF OREGON CENTRAL MILITARY RD.

To VIEWPOINT

MIDDLE FORK WILLAMETTE RIVER

CAMPSITE
VAULT TOILETS
WATER

GETTING THERE

From Oakridge (about 40 miles southeast of Eugene on SR 58), turn right on Kitson Springs Road, just east of town. Go 0.5 miles, and turn right on FS 21 (also known as Rigdon Road and Diamond Drive). Travel 26 miles to the campground, on your right.

McKenzie River and SR 126 (see Frissell Crossing, page 11, for more information on the Aufderheide).

Closer to the Oakridge end of FS 21, an alternative camping option, Larison Cove, is a canoe-in day-use area on a 1.5-mile-long arm of Hills Creek Reservoir, where motorized boats are prohibited. Two picnic tables and fire rings sit there in a quiet old-growth setting, and dispersed camping is available in the area. A Northwest Forest Pass is required to park at the put-in, which is at FS 2106, after about 3 miles on FS 21. You'll also find a vault toilet and garbage service at the put-in.

GPS COORDINATES

UTM Zone (WGS84)   10T
Easting   0554250
Northing   4816160
Latitude   N 43.4964°
Longitude   W 122.329°

44
THIELSEN VIEW CAMPGROUND

THIELSEN VIEW IS ONE OF SEVERAL Forest Service campgrounds in the Diamond Lake vicinity, but it's removed from the mayhem of SR 138 because it sits alone on the western shore. With two other campgrounds across scenic Diamond Lake that can accommodate several hundred campers between them, chances are you won't find yourself alone out in this seemingly remote territory.

Diamond Lake is an immensely popular area, particularly for trout fishermen who troll the lake's crystalline waters for their share of the plentiful rainbows (the lake is stocked with 450,000 fingerlings annually). The lake's name comes from the abundance of glassy volcanic rock that litters this region of Umpqua National Forest.

Great fishing notwithstanding, Diamond Lake's popularity can be attributed to a number of other factors. For starters, Diamond Lake is one of the largest natural lakes in Oregon. Add to this its proximity to some spectacular mountain scenery. Follow that up with blissfully warm, dry summer weather. The place is also a convenient distance north of Crater Lake National Park (where frightening numbers of visitors gather in any given summer) and quickly absorbs the overflow. Last but not least, the drive from Roseburg off I-5 follows the pristine and picturesque North Umpqua River most of the way to Diamond Lake on SR 138. This stretch of highway has been called one of the prettiest drives in western America in the summertime, and it is also one of the main connectors between western and eastern Oregon. All of these factors add up to plenty of people most of the time.

A sizable share of the wonder at Diamond Lake comes in the form of snowy, knife-like mountain peaks— Mount Bailey to the west and, as the campground name implies, Mount Thielsen to the east. Both will take

> *The lone campground on the western shore of Diamond Lake has views galore and a multitude of recreational options.*

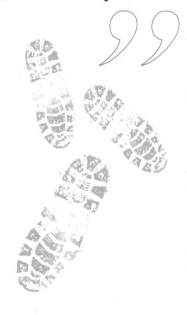

RATINGS

Beauty: ✪ ✪ ✪ ✪ ✪
Privacy: ✪ ✪ ✪ ✪
Spaciousness: ✪ ✪ ✪ ✪ ✪
Quiet: ✪ ✪ ✪ ✪ ✪
Security: ✪ ✪ ✪ ✪
Cleanliness: ✪ ✪ ✪ ✪ ✪
Insect control: ✪ ✪ ✪

KEY INFORMATION

ADDRESS: Thielsen View
Campground
c/o Diamond Lake
Ranger District
2020 Toketee
Ranger Station
Road
Idleyld Park, OR
97447

OPERATED BY: Umpqua National
Forest

INFORMATION: (541) 498-2515

OPEN: Mid-May–mid-
October, depend-
ing on snow level

SITES: 60

EACH SITE: Picnic table, fire
grill

ASSIGNMENT: First come,
first served; no
reservations

REGISTRATION: Self-registration
on site

FACILITIES: Vault toilets,
piped water,
garbage service,
boat ramp

PARKING: At campsites

FEE: $11; $4 per additional vehicle

ELEVATION: 5,190 feet

RESTRICTIONS: *Pets:* On leash only
Fires: In fire grills
only
Alcohol: Permitted
Vehicles: 24-foot
RV size limit,
no hookups
Other: 14-day stay
limit

some time to explore, since the only way to fully appreciate them is by foot over arduous trails full of loose, crumbling pumice. The rock is modern-day evidence of the eruption of Mount Mazama some 6,700 years ago.

The upper portion of 9,182-foot Mount Thielsen is a technical climb and should be attempted only by those with the appropriate skills and equipment. Less difficult hikes abound, however, throughout Umpqua National Forest, Mount Thielsen Wilderness, and Oregon Cascades Recreation Area, all within access of Thielsen View Campground. Mount Thielsen Wilderness alone has roughly 125 miles of hiking trails, including a 30-mile section of the Pacific Crest National Scenic Trail. Easier trails in the region range from the 3.2-mile ramble to Horse and Teal Lakes (accessed from the South Shore picnic area) to the longer but still gentle Rodney Butte Trail (6.4 miles roundtrip). A bit steeper challenge awaits on the Tipsoo Trail, which switchbacks for an elevation gain of 1,500 feet to a spectacular vista, and the Howlock Mountain Trail, which is difficult but connects to the Pacific Crest Trail after 7 miles.

Hiking, however, doesn't become an option at the higher elevations much before July, when the heavy snowfalls of winter melt from the trails. In the meantime and at various times throughout the year, there's mountain biking along Forest Service roads and designated trails (except in wilderness areas). For a full-circle look at the area and to get warmed up to more strenuous activity, try the paved bike paths that circle Diamond Lake. Other options are angling in nearby creeks, hunting, birdwatching, canoeing and kayaking the North Umpqua River, and lowland walks to Lemolo Falls and Toketee Falls. If nothing else, there's sitting in camp and enjoying the incredibly clear mountain air.

The approach of winter doesn't slow down activity much in the Diamond Lake area. Although the campground is closed, the resort on the east shore of the lake is the focal point for a myriad of skiing and snowmobiling options. At Mount Bailey, you can get in a half-dozen exhilarating runs on pristine powder (considered the best in the state) via a privately run snowcat system. There's a Nordic ski center at Diamond Lake

MAP

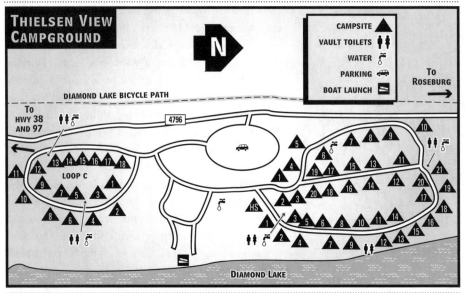

Resort complete with rentals and groomed trails. For the snowmobiler there is a plethora of trails, short or long, guided or on your own. You can ride as far Crater Lake to the south or Crescent Lake to the north (the latter a full-day roundtrip of eight hours).

GETTING THERE

From Roseburg and I-5, take SR 138 to Clearwater (about 50 miles southeast), where the road leaves the North Umpqua and parallels Clearwater River. Turn right onto FS 4795 (Diamond Lake Loop), and head around the north end of Diamond Lake 3.3 miles to Thielsen View Campground on the left. From Medford, take US 62 north to SR 230 north, then continue to SR 138. At FS 4795, turn left and proceed as above. From Klamath Falls or Bend, take US 97 and follow the signs to Diamond Lake Recreation Area.

GPS COORDINATES

UTM Zone (WGS84)   10T
Easting   0567629
Northing   4779951
Latitude   N 43.1693°
Longitude   W 122.168°

> *An exquisite tent-camping setting on the spine of the Cascades with hiking options in all directions.*

THIS LITTLE GEM IS THE SOURCE of the Middle Fork Willamette River and sits within the Oregon Cascades Recreation Area (OCRA) about as close to the spine of the Cascade Range as you can get without leaving western Oregon. You can practically smell the juniper when the wind blows from the east.

My introduction to Timpanogas came at the end of a long, hot day over rough roads and with a fair amount of backtracking—hazards of the job, I'm afraid—but my nerves were shot and my patience was rice-paper thin. Maybe it was this fragile combination, but when I crested the knoll that gave me my first glimpse of Timpanogas Lake and the campground, I wept. Honest! If they had been auctioning off building sites around the lake right then and there, I would have sold my body and soul.

After spending weeks on the research trail and developing a keen snobbery for tent camping, I could quickly recognize a keeper when I saw one. First of all, they're so damned rare. And, secondly, you usually find them when you least expect it. Pleasant surprises are still shocking, you know.

I made a fast run through the campground loop, then parked near site #1. I was in a daze for about the first 15 minutes as I digested the exquisite setting that lay before me. I almost didn't want to move for fear it would disappear in a poof!

Let me describe the scene, and you can make your own assessment: The faint but distinctive chirping of an eagle carried across the water from its perch high in the forest of firs bordering the lake. A bright red canoe slid into view from the periphery of the lake, contrasting pleasantly with the deep blue water and the rich green forest. A bold chipmunk scratched around nervously under the picnic table, hoping I had brought new and interesting forage. Songbirds flitted everywhere. Waterfowl bobbed along the water's edge. The

RATINGS

Beauty: ✿ ✿ ✿
Privacy: ✿ ✿ ✿ ✿
Spaciousness: ✿ ✿ ✿ ✿
Quiet: ✿ ✿ ✿ ✿ ✿
Security: ✿ ✿ ✿
Cleanliness: ✿ ✿ ✿
Insect control: ✿ ✿ ✿

fragrance of an early evening campfire mixed with the warm mountain scents of a late afternoon sun.

How are we doing so far? Idyllic, you say? Absolutely. This is prototypical Timpanogas, and I hope it never changes. You know what they say. First impressions are lasting.

The campground itself is an elegantly simplistic collection of sites, all but two of which claim "low-bank waterfront" and "private moorage" in their brochure descriptions. The two vanguards (sites 1 and 7) can at least claim "territorial views" of the lake or the surrounding campground. There isn't one site that doesn't have what real-estate agents call "curb appeal". Each sits on practically a full-sized city lot and if you get to "own" site 9 for a few days, you'll have the best claim to pumped-water rights.

Conversely, site 5 sits at an awkward distance from the water spigot on the spur road to the Timpanogas Basin (Indigo Lake) trailhead, which requires the Northwest Forest Pass. Not to be outdone, however, it features the most shaded setting under a high crown of varietal firs. Thick underbrush otherwise maintains maximum privacy between sites along the camp road and tree cover is just enough to allow for filtered sun in some places, direct blasts in others. The sites are so spaciously distant from each other, however, that lack of privacy is hardly a consideration. It's the kind of community intimate as it may seem—where you can choose to meet your neighbors or not.

Maybe it's the high altitude (5,200 feet) and the achingly fresh air that energizes your sense of discovery at Timpanogas. Maybe it's the ghostly presence of pioneers who stalwartly clambered with their cumbersome wagons and ox teams over the Cascades at nearby Emigrant Pass. Maybe it's the call of the Pacific Crest National Scenic Trail, which passes a few miles east.

Whatever the inspiration, a restlessness sets in at Timpanogas once the initial shock of such a pleasant place has passed. More than 25 trail miles connect within the Timpanogas Basin alone, leading to such delights as Opal Lake, Indigo Lake (with a hike-in campsite), June Lake, and politically incorrect Amos and Andy Lakes. Views in all directions are possible

KEY INFORMATION

ADDRESS:	Timpanogas Lake Campground c/o Middle Fork Ranger District 46375 OR 58 Westfir, OR 97492
OPERATED BY:	Willamette National Forest
INFORMATION:	(541) 782-2283
OPEN:	July–October, depending on snow level
SITES:	10
EACH SITE:	Picnic table, fire grill, some shade trees
ASSIGNMENT:	First come, first served; no reservations
REGISTRATION:	Self-registration on site
FACILITIES:	Vault toilets, piped water, garbage service
PARKING:	At campsites
FEE:	$8; $4 per additional vehicle
ELEVATION:	5,200 feet
RESTRICTIONS:	*Pets:* On leash only *Fires:* In fire pits only *Alcohol:* Permitted *Vehicles:* 24-foot RV size limit, no hookups *Other:* 14-day stay limit

MAP

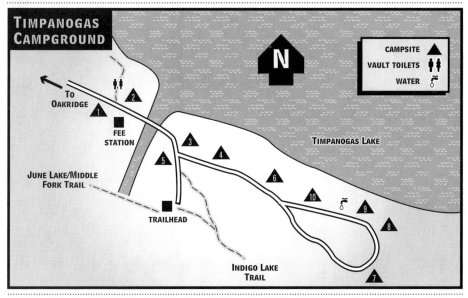

TIMPANOGAS CAMPGROUND

CAMPSITE
VAULT TOILETS
WATER

N

To OAKRIDGE

FEE STATION

JUNE LAKE/MIDDLE FORK TRAIL

TRAILHEAD

TIMPANOGAS LAKE

INDIGO LAKE TRAIL

GETTING THERE

Timpanogas Lake is 43 miles southeast of Oakridge by way of the following route: From OR 58 2 miles east of Oakridge, take Kitson Springs Road (FS 23) south briefly to its intersection with FS 21 (alternately known in spots as Rigdon Road and Military Road). Turn right on FS 21, passing Hills Creek Reservoir and numerous campgrounds—including Sacandaga—and along the Middle Fork Willamette River roughly 32 miles to FS 2154. Turn left, and follow the road 10 miles to the campground. Stretches of FS 2154 are rough and steep as the elevation gain is rapid as you approach 5,200 feet.

from certain trail vantage points, with Sawtooth Mountain to the south, Cowhorn Mountain (at 7,664 feet, the highest point in the OCRA) to the east, and Diamond Peak to the north. The same Middle Fork Willamette River Trail that passes by Sacandaga Campground (see page 139) ends at Timpanogas Lake and is a 25-mile one-way trek along the river's banks and parts of the Central Military Wagon Road.

Wintertime activities in the OCRA are gaining in popularity, namely snowmobiling (since the recreation designation allows for semi-primitive motorized use) and cross-country skiing. Fair warning: mosquitoes are said to be pretty bad here in July and early August. Something about dogs being carried off . . .

GPS COORDINATES

UTM Zone (WGS84)   10T
Easting   0571653
Northing   4806749
Latitude   N 43.4102°
Longitude   W 122.115°

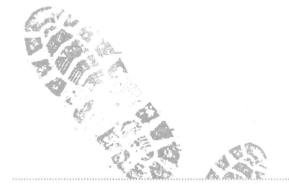

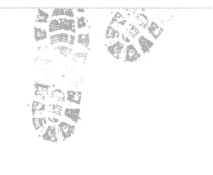

SOUTHERN **COAST**

IF YOU'RE LOOKING FOR A QUIET, fairly small, and rather quaint camping area close to the central Oregon Coast but just a few miles from the busy coastal US 101, then Canal Creek is an excellent spot for a night or two.

Canal Creek Campground is located in the lush Siuslaw National Forest. Open all year with easy drive-to access, one could describe it as a "nice little campground." It consists of one circular camping area and one group area. There are 11 drive-in sites in the first section and a large grassy field for open camping in the group section. It is my understanding that if the group camping area is not reserved, which is often the case, then non-groups can camp there.

Nestled in a steep canyon carved out by Canal Creek, the lush campground is home to large fern bushes, waxmyrtle, blackberries and huckleberries under a canopy of Douglas fir and spruce. True to its name, a very nice 20-foot-wide rippling creek encircles both sections of the camp. In fact, Canal Creek divides one side from the other. No need to fret, though, as Forest Service staff have thought of everything, including a 30-foot walking bridge spanning the creek and connecting the two areas. There is an inconspicuous road through the creek to the group camp, but it is only usable during the drier summer season.

Each campsite in the first section has drive-in parking, a fire pit, and a picnic table. The group section has a large fire pit and picnic tables, usually kept under the covered shelter, and a 300-foot-diameter grassy area. There is a large covered shelter with seating located just over the footbridge near the group camp section. Not surprisingly, given that Camp Creek is a Forest Service campground, there aren't showers, but there are adequate, though not flush, toilets and an old-fashioned hand pump for fresh water—just like at

> *Here's a year-round option in the Siuslaw National Forest with easy access to coastal and wilderness areas.*

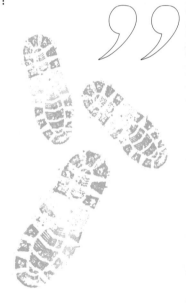

RATINGS

Beauty: ✿ ✿ ✿ ✿
Privacy: ✿ ✿ ✿
Spaciousness: ✿ ✿ ✿ ✿
Quiet: ✿ ✿ ✿ ✿
Security: ✿ ✿ ✿
Cleanliness: ✿ ✿ ✿
Insect Control: ✿ ✿

KEY INFORMATION

ADDRESS: Canal Creek Campground c/o Waldport Ranger District P. O. Box 400 Waldport, OR 97394

OPERATED BY: American Land and Leisure for Suislaw National Forest

INFORMATION: (541) 547-3679

RESERVATIONS: (877) 444-6777 (toll-free)

OPEN: Year-round

SITES: 11

EACH SITE: Picnic table, fire ring

ASSIGNMENT: First come, first served; reservations for group camp only

REGISTRATION: Self-registration on site

FACILITIES: Vault toilets, hand-pumped water (April–September), garbage service, group site with picnic shelter and play field

PARKING: At sites only

FEE: $17; group site (1–50 people) $115; group site (51–100 people) $165; winter rates are reduced and posted

ELEVATION: Sea level

RESTRICTIONS: *Pets:* On leash only *Fires:* In fire rings only *Alcohol:* Permitted *Vehicles:* 2 vehicles per site; small RVs possible

Grandma's. Everybody in the park meets at the water pump sooner or later to exchange (and possibly expand) adventure stories, stir up a little gossip, or maybe even spark a romance. Stranger things have happened . . .

From the coastal town of Waldport on US 101, you need to hang to the left (east) immediately at the south end of the famous Alsea Bay bridge. This puts you on the Alsea Highway. East exactly 7 miles (yep, no more, no less), you will find the sign for Canal Creek Campground with an arrow directing you 4 miles up FS 3462. If you ever wondered what it is like driving around the south island of New Zealand, then this is your road. Nicely paved, though narrow, it winds and winds and winds in a comical back and forth way. With the slow going, you'll have a chance to be impressed with the vast number of bushy green ferns hanging on the sheer ridge wall along the road. Pretty impressive, especially if fern grottoes are your thing.

If you venture out and about on the coast, there is much to do, from beach walks to fishing to bay crabbing. For a few bucks, you can have a great afternoon of fun by renting several crab rings with bait and crabbing off the Waldport public pier, located off the Alsea Highway on the east end of town. Only 9 miles south from Waldport on US 101 is the coastal town of Yachats, which is the number one place in the United States for wild mushrooms. Numerous shops and the visitor center have information on great hikes as well as places to look for mushrooms. (Remember, if you aren't sure, consider all mushrooms poisonous). The Drift Creek Wilderness is not far from Canal Creek Campground on the north side of Alsea Highway, accessible via FS 3446. This small but wondrous little preserve has claim to the largest stand of old-growth forest remaining in the Coast Range. A must-see, in my estimation.

The Alsea River is most known for steelhead and salmon fishing in the fall & winter. It's a good river for beginning and intermediate paddlers (during the summer), as it has few technical rapids. Log snags can be the most significant hazard along with drifting logs, so be on the lookout if you go paddling.

MAP

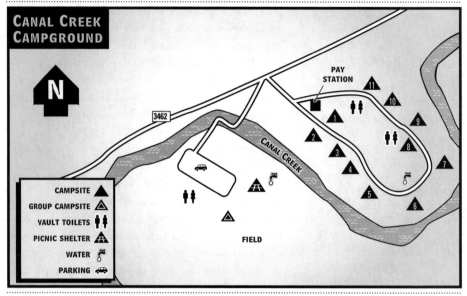

CANAL CREEK
CAMPGROUND

N

PAY STATION

3462

CANAL CREEK

CAMPSITE
GROUP CAMPSITE
VAULT TOILETS
PICNIC SHELTER
WATER
PARKING

FIELD

GETTING THERE

From Waldport on US 101, veer left at the south end of Waldport Bridge onto the Alsea Highway (OR 34). Continue 7 miles before turning at the campground sign onto the access road, FS 3462. From Albany in the Willamette Valley, head west on US 20 through Corvallis (OR 34 picks up US 20 here) for 15 miles to Philomath. Stay left on OR 34 (Alsea Highway) when it splits from US 20, and continue 52 very winding miles (most along the Alsea River) to FS 3462. Turn left, and Canal Creek Campground is 4 miles in on paved road.

GPS COORDINATES

UTM Zone (WGS84)	10T
Easting	0425990
Northing	4914066
Latitude	N 44.3761°
Longitude	W 123.929°

47
CAPE BLANCO STATE PARK CAMPGROUND

> *Cape Blanco is the westernmost point in Oregon and home to the most westerly lighthouse (historic Cape Blanco Light) on the United States mainland.*

WESTWARD TO US 101 and down the coast, we encounter our second installment in the cape collection (for the others, see pages 113and 156). While the entire Oregon Coast is one long necklace of windswept headlands and craggy contours linked by a glistening thread of lowland sand dunes and tidal waterways, Capes Blanco, Lookout, and Perpetua are particularly stunning for their natural visual appeal, recreational opportunity, and geologic wonder.

Cape Blanco State Park is the farthest south. The cape, park, reef, lighthouse, airport, and road from US 101 all bear the name Blanco, first given to the dramatic ivory cliffs that rise 200 feet above a black sand beach. In 1603, a relatively unknown Spanish explorer named Martin d'Aguilar spotted the sheer white ("blanco," to him) cliffs and aptly dubbed them for posterity.

This state park covers 1,895 acres of forested headlands and wildflower fields, which flood the area with color in late spring and early summer. Yellow coneflowers, coral bells, yellow sand verbena, and northern dune tansy are the most prevalent varieties. Sitka spruce dominates in the tree department. Farther east in the coastal mountain ranges, one can find old-growth Douglas fir and the commercially prized Port Orford cedar.

The lush vegetation that stays green all year at Cape Blanco (thanks to the temperate marine climate) has been thoughtfully preserved in the campground, lending a certain air of mystery to many of the campsites. If you are lucky enough to snag one that backs up to the ocean, you'll have a thick forest as your buffer for the ultimate in tent-camping privacy. Surprisingly, considering how close the campground sits to the ocean, none seem to have water views. Only two of the cabins are situated to take in any views of the ocean, but it's only a short walk to the bluff for a panoramic

RATINGS

Beauty: ✩ ✩ ✩ ✩ ✩
Privacy: ✩ ✩ ✩
Spaciousness: ✩ ✩ ✩ ✩
Quiet: ✩ ✩ ✩ (summer)
✩ ✩ ✩ ✩ ✩ (winter)
Security: ✩ ✩ ✩ ✩
Cleanliness: ✩ ✩ ✩ ✩ ✩
Insect Control: ✩ ✩ ✩

vista. In a thick fog, however, make sure you know where the bluff ends and that unplanned shortcut to the beach starts! Heavy fog can prevail anytime between late October and May, but it's between December and February that the rains make their mark on Cape Blanco—and in generous supply. More than half of the area's total annual rainfall occurs in this three-month stretch. Summers (thank heavens) are generally sunny and mild. Temperatures are rarely extremely hot or cold. Shoulder seasons (March–April and September–October) bring a mixture of warm, cool, drizzly, breezy, sunny, and cloudy weather. And that's just in one day!

These shoulder seasons (part of "The Discovery Season," as it's called by Oregon State Parks and Recreation) can be the perfect time to enjoy a place like Cape Blanco. The summer tourist season along the Oregon Coast—all 360 miles of it—is lovely weather-wise, and the scenery is consistently spectacular, but high season is nevertheless an experience you could learn to hate. There is little relief from the crowds, campgrounds fill up quickly (including Cape Blanco, which doesn't require reservations), and the main north–south route (US 101) is one long, nearly unbroken procession of RVs and trailers.

But if summer is the only time you can get there, by all means go. You just have to be a little more creative to find the pockets of isolation. Joining the seals offshore in the string of craggy, black basalt outcroppings of Oregon Islands National Wildlife Refuge may be a bit extreme, however. That's what binoculars are for. Instead, try the New River paddle route just upcoast from the park in the town of Denmark. This 8-mile stretch of tidewater attracts shorebirds and migratory waterfowl. The New River is a blend of fresh waters descending from Coast Ranges and the salty Pacific, creating an interesting mix of plant and animal life. On one end of the river is undeveloped Floras Lake State Park, and at the other end are the sand dunes of Bandon. Both are equally worthy of exploration.

Another alternative is the Sixes River, which forms the northern boundary of Cape Blanco State Park. Fishing in the Sixes is best in the off-season: chinook in the fall, sea-run cutthroat trout in spring and

KEY INFORMATION

ADDRESS:	Cape Blanco State Park 39745 S. US 101 Port Orford, OR 97465
OPERATED BY:	Oregon State Parks
INFORMATION:	(541) 332-6774; www.oregon stateparks.org
OPEN:	Year-round
SITES:	53 with electric and water, separate hiker/biker camp
EACH SITE:	Picnic table, fire grill, electricity, some shade trees; hiker/biker camp has no electricity
ASSIGNMENT:	First come, first served; no reservations
REGISTRATION:	On site
FACILITIES:	Bathhouse with sinks, toilets, hot showers; firewood; laundry; some disabled access; 4 reservable rustic log cabins, $35; reservable group camp (30–50) and horse camp
PARKING:	At campsites
FEE:	Electric sites $16 May–September, $12 October–April; hiker/biker sites $4 May–September and free October–April; $5 per additional vehicle
ELEVATION:	200 feet
RESTRICTIONS:	*Pets:* On leash only *Fires:* In fire pits *Alcohol:* Prohibited *Vehicles:* No limit *Other:* 14-day stay limit

MAP

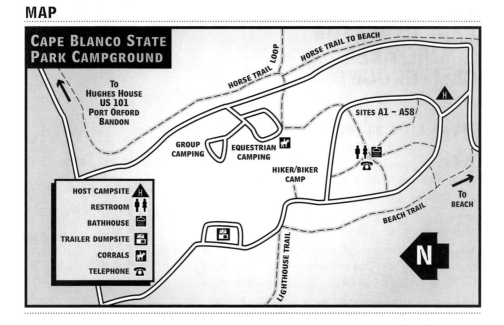

CAPE BLANCO STATE PARK CAMPGROUND

To
HUGHES HOUSE
US 101
PORT ORFORD
BANDON

HORSE TRAIL LOOP

HORSE TRAIL TO BEACH

SITES A1 – A58

GROUP CAMPING

EQUESTRIAN CAMPING

HIKER/BIKER CAMP

To BEACH

BEACH TRAIL

LIGHTHOUSE TRAIL

HOST CAMPSITE
RESTROOM
BATHHOUSE
TRAILER DUMPSITE
CORRALS
TELEPHONE

N

GETTING THERE

To reach Cape Blanco State Park from Port Orford, drive north on US 101 to Cape Blanco Highway, and then go 5 miles west to the campground.

GPS COORDINATES

UTM Zone (WGS84)   10T
Easting   0373316
Northing   4743269
Latitude   N 42.8315°
Longitude   W 124.55°

fall, and steelhead in the winter. There are several boat put-ins along the river east of US 101. Hikers can take their pick of varying topographies. A moderate climb up to the windswept bluff near the lighthouse offers views in all directions: north to Blacklock Point and Tower Rock, west across Blanco Reef, and south to Orford Reef. This is an excellent vantage point from which to watch gray whales on their migration path from the Arctic to Baja, California, in winter months.

Down on the beach, you can walk along portions of the Oregon Coast Trail, but keep in mind that tide levels change anywhere from 6 to 12 feet twice daily. The ultimate escape for those experienced enough to handle it is Grassy Knob Wilderness, which lies not far east in a small section of Siskiyou National Forest. Backpacking through this area is best described as bushwhacking; there are very few established trails and the going is steep and rugged.

48
CAPE PERPETUA SCENIC AREA CAMPGROUND

CAPE **PERPETUA, THE LAST OF THE CAPE TRIO,** was named by Captain James Cook in 1778. Cook passed by as he fearlessly continued north on his fruitless search for the Pacific link to the Northwest Passage. Both Cape Perpetua and the nearby town of Yachats (pronounced "yah-hots") have long been favored vacation destinations for Oregonians who appreciate the small town's relative seclusion amidst some of the coast's most awe-inspiring scenery. For some unknown reason, Yachats is often overlooked by tourists heading for the bustling centers of Newport and Florence, nearly equidistant to the north and south respectively.

Long before tourists had a road to take them anywhere in this vicinity, however, the fog-shrouded seashore and mountain slopes were the domain of coastal Indian tribes who fished, clammed, and hunted in blissful obscurity. Their contentment was short-lived once the Spanish, English, and Germans discovered the rich resources in the area. Along the coast and up nearby verdant river valleys, timber mills, fish canneries, and dairy farms thrived from the late-eighteenth century through the twentieth. While there is still significant activity in these traditional industries, tourism has begun to replace them in the last several decades. Waning resources have forced residents of towns and villages all along the Oregon coast to consider alternative methods of making a living. The transition has not been easy for many of them.

While tourism has only recently seen dramatic growth, the makings for a tourism boom were first put in place in the 1930s with the extension of US 101 and the construction of the first Cape Perpetua Visitor Center by the Civilian Conservation Corps. Today's center is a renovated version of the original, and there is still evidence of the Depression-era workers' housing on the trail between the center and the beach.

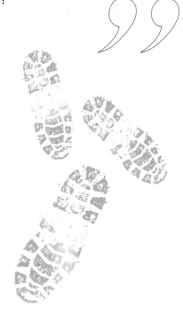

> *Cape Perpetua is widely considered to be one of the Oregon coast's most spectacular headlands.*

RATINGS

Beauty: ✿ ✿ ✿ ✿ ✿
Privacy: ✿ ✿
Spaciousness: ✿ ✿ ✿
Quiet: ✿ ✿ ✿ ✿
Security: ✿ ✿ ✿ ✿
Cleanliness: ✿ ✿ ✿ ✿
Insect Control: ✿ ✿ ✿ ✿

KEY INFORMATION

ADDRESS:	Cape Perpetua Scenic Area 2400 US 101 Yachats, OR 97498
OPERATED BY:	American Land and Leisure for Siuslaw National Forest
INFORMATION:	(541) 547-3289
OPEN:	Mid-May–late September
SITES:	38
EACH SITE:	Picnic table, fire grill
ASSIGNMENT:	Reservations online at www .recreation.gov or by phone at (877) 444-6777
REGISTRATION:	Self-registration on site
FACILITIES:	Flush toilets, piped water, sanitation station, group camp, public telephone at visitor center
PARKING:	At campsites (back-in parking recommended)
FEE:	$20; plus $5 per additional vehicle
ELEVATION:	Just above sea level
RESTRICTIONS:	*Pets:* On leash only *Fires:* In fire pits only *Alcohol:* Permitted *Vehicles:* RVs up to 22 feet

The center is a good starting point before taking in the sights of this unique area. As the focal point of the surrounding piece of land known as the Cape Perpetua Scenic Area, the center offers educational exhibits and films as well as a small bookshop. Trails from the center lead off into stands of old-growth spruce in one direction and under the highway to the beach in another. All in all, there are 22 miles of hiking trails within the scenic area. Flanked by state parks on its north and south sides, a wilderness area on the east, the highly photogenic Heceta Head Lighthouse not far south, and the famed Stellar Sea Lion Caves just beyond that, Cape Perpetua Scenic Area has no lack of interesting day trips for visitors based at the campground.

Ah yes, the campground. Cape Perpetua Campground is actually two camping areas within the jurisdiction of the Siuslaw National Forest (as is the rest of the scenic area) but managed by a private contractor, American Lands and Leisure. Both are quite close to the visitor center, and the only difference between them is that one is an individual-site complex and the other accommodates groups of up to 50 people. Privacy at the individual-site campground is less than ideal. To be honest, I contemplated eliminating this entry from the revised book, but after canvassing alternative parks and campgrounds up and down the coast, I decided to stick with Cape Perpetua. Although privacy is painfully lacking because the sites are stretched out along the access road with little vegetation between them, at least they are situated between a creek and a cape so as to give the feeling of being tucked away. Most other campgrounds in the immediate area are sprawling compounds that easily defy description as peaceful.

The campground operates mid-May to late September, but it's worth mentioning that the wild and windswept Cape Perpetua is an enormously popular whale-watching spot in the wintertime. Although the campgrounds are not open, the visitor center has interpretive programs for the whale-watching crowd.

If you want to witness prime examples of the geologic magnificence found at Cape Perpetua Scenic Area close up, stop at Devil's Churn and Captain Cook's Chasm. The relentless movement of sea against basalt

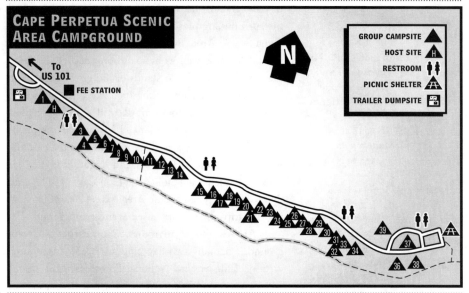

CAPE PERPETUA SCENIC AREA CAMPGROUND

To US 101

FEE STATION

N

GROUP CAMPSITE
HOST SITE
RESTROOM
PICNIC SHELTER
TRAILER DUMPSITE

rock has formed overhanging cliffs and caves, which are pounded mercilessly at high tides by clashing currents that explode as high as 60 feet into the air. The effect is exhilarating.

All along this portion of the sculpted coast is an endless array of rugged inlets, crescent-shaped coves, and towering capes. Just south of Devil's Churn is the road up to the Cape Perpetua Viewpoint. At 800 feet above the sea, you can have a bird's-eye view of this breathtaking panorama in all directions.

GETTING THERE

To reach Cape Perpetua from Yachats (23 miles south of Newport), drive 3 miles south on US 101. The park entrance is on the non-ocean side.

GPS COORDINATES

UTM Zone (WGS84)   10T
Easting   0411669
Northing   4903835
Latitude   N 44.2824°
Longitude   W 124.107°

> *Backed against some of the largest dunes in Oregon Dunes National Recreation Area, Eel Creek affords a stunning and unforgettable outdoor experience.*

WELCOME TO THE HEART OF Oregon Dunes National Recreation Area. If you've never ventured into this stunning sector of the Oregon coast, prepare yourself for an experience that you will not forget.

Eel Creek is just one of many campgrounds that are clustered in the Florence/Reedsport/Coos Bay stretch of US 101. Aside from its vegetation-lush private sites, Eel Creek's strongest selling point is the absence of off-road vehicle access to the dunes.

Why these noisy machines are allowed in a place of such serene and fragile beauty is beyond me. Fortunately there are 32,000 acres of sand in the National Recreation Area, and the jeep trail stops short a mile or two south of Eel Creek, so there's space for everyone here. If you want peace and quiet as part of your dunes experience, however, make sure to avoid hiking in an area where they rent dune buggies.

Eel Creek backs up against some of the largest dunes in the 46-mile-long protected beach. Always shifting, always changing, some dunes reach as high as 600 feet. Slog your way to the top of one of these monsters and look out over a most spectacular sight—sand, sand, and more sand. Swirled and sculpted in some places, smoothed and glistening like satin in others, rising and falling like patterns of the sea frozen in motion, the pale undulations radiate under a startlingly blue August sky.

The Pacific Ocean is solely responsible for these magnificent mounds, starting some 13,000 years ago when glacial sediment first began the tireless task of forming this section of Oregon's coast. Since then, rivers flowing out of the nearby Coast Range have also contributed their share of deposits. Seasonal patterns of wind and waves combine to add their influence to the sand's destiny, making these the largest collection of active, or "living," coastal sand dunes in America.

RATINGS

Beauty: ✿ ✿ ✿ ✿ ✿
Privacy: ✿ ✿ ✿ ✿ ✿
Spaciousness: ✿ ✿ ✿ ✿
Quiet: ✿ ✿ ✿ ✿ ✿
Security: ✿ ✿ ✿ ✿
Cleanliness: ✿ ✿ ✿ ✿
Insect Control: ✿ ✿ ✿

Believe it or not, from Eel Creek Campground due west to the ocean is roughly 2 miles. There are places in Oregon Dunes National Recreation Area where the dunes are as much as 3 miles wide—a stiff distance when you're making your way through soft sand. The easiest way to traverse the dunes is along any of the 30 hiking trails within the Recreation Area. It is best to keep to the trails for more noble reasons as well. This is a highly fragile ecosystem, with more than 400 different wildlife species inhabiting the dunes. Of these, 175 are birds.

Headquarters for Oregon Dunes National Recreation Area is right on US 101 at the junction with SR 38 in Reedsport. This is a well-stocked information bureau, with plenty of free guides, brochures, maps, and assorted publications. The exhibits are worth a look, too. It's also a good place to compare notes with other travelers.

As with many other parts of western Oregon, late summer and early fall are prime times, weatherwise, for enjoying the dunes at their best. If it's any indication of winter conditions, Reedsport holds an annual Storm Festival in February. Wind speeds have been clocked as high as 100 miles an hour. Generally, the wind is more problematic than rain. Even in summer, clear skies and warm temperatures are tempered by incessant offshore breezes that often kick up little flurries of sand, which playfully tickle the ankles but can be aggravating at eye level. Sand inside a camera body can be ruinous and costly, so protect your equipment.

Aside from the mesmerizing appeal of the dunes, you'll find a variety of other attractions. The Winchester Bay area offers guided and chartered fishing options, clamming spots too numerous to mention, and a museum and lighthouse. Inland along the Umpqua River is Dean Creek Elk Viewing Area, a 923-acre preserve for free-roaming Roosevelt elk, which are native to the area. The spot also attracts a multitude of waterfowl and migratory birds, including osprey, bald eagles, and blue herons.

It's easy to confuse this campground with Mid Eel, which is only minutes away. Watch for signs to Eel Creek Campground about 12 miles south of Reedsport.

KEY INFORMATION

ADDRESS: Eel Creek Campground Oregon Dunes National Recreation Area 855 US 101 Reedsport, OR 97467

OPERATED BY: Northwest Land Management for Siuslaw National Forest

INFORMATION: (541) 271-6000

OPEN: Mid-May–mid-September

SITES: 52

EACH SITE: Picnic table, fire grill

ASSIGNMENT: First come, first served; or by reservation in summer at (877) 444-6777 or www .recreation.gov

REGISTRATION: Self-registration on site or at camp host

FACILITIES: Flush toilets, drinking water, boat launch and rentals at nearby Eel Lake

PARKING: At campsites

FEE: $20; $5 each additional vehicle

ELEVATION: Sea level

RESTRICTIONS: *Pets:* On leash only *Fires:* In fire pits only *Alcohol:* Permitted *Vehicles:* RVs and trailers up to 35 feet

MAP

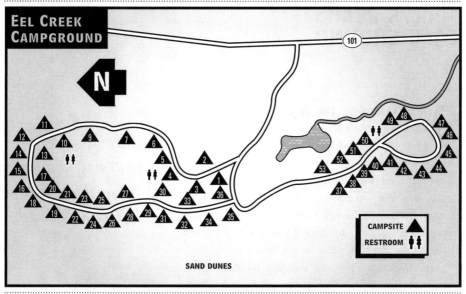

GETTING THERE

From Reedsport, drive south on US 101 for 12 miles. The campground entrance is on the ocean side.

The campground is right off US 101 but surprisingly quiet given its close proximity to a busy thoroughfare. Heavy vegetation helps absorb traffic sounds and provides lovely secluded, sandy-bottomed tent sites. Ocean breezes help keep insects to a minimum.

GPS COORDINATES

UTM Zone (WGS84)   10T
Easting   0404377
Northing   4826685
Latitude   N 43.587°
Longitude   W 124.1845°

MARYS PEAK CAMPGROUND

ON A CLEAR DAY, THE VIEWS from atop Marys Peak are unparalleled. Mount Rainier is visible to the north, Mount Hood to the east, and Mount Jefferson to the southeast. The Alsea River, favored by fishermen from the Corvallis/Eugene area for its bountiful steelhead, fall chinook, and coho salmon, fans out to the west with the glistening Pacific beyond. The Alsea is just one of a dozen major rivers sliding out of the Coast Range and into the Pacific.

At 4,097 feet, you are standing on the highest point in the Oregon Coast Range. Sir Edmund Hillary would have to be slightly amused at the modest elevation, but even he could appreciate that undeniable exhilaration of knowing that you are looking down on everything for as far as the eye can see.

Marys Peak (and all of the Coast Range for that matter) sits on ancient basalt that was part of the Pacific Ocean floor some 50 to 60 million years ago. Constant uplifting and shifting of tectonic plates pushes the mountain range ever upward, although the evidence of this activity is not as easily seen on Marys Peak as elsewhere in the range. The dense forest and thick mulchy soil obscure geologic evidence, making this one of the toughest areas for geologists to examine accurately.

If you are familiar with Coast Range weather, you will know that cloudless days on Marys Peak are rare indeed. Siuslaw National Forest, within which Marys Peak is located, is a coastal rain forest. That should give you some idea of the degree of wetness that pervades the place. The average annual rainfall in Siuslaw is 90 inches. There are normally as many as 180 days of measurable precipitation annually.

The driest times are late summer and early fall. Don't rule out wintertime, which can actually be quite fun when a substantial snowfall covers the peak and makes it an ideal, untracked wonderland for cross-

> *This intimate, tents-only campground sits at the highest point in Oregon's Coast.*

RATINGS

Beauty: ✩ ✩ ✩ ✩
Privacy: ✩ ✩ ✩
Spaciousness: ✩ ✩ ✩
Quiet: ✩ ✩ ✩ ✩ ✩
Security: ✩ ✩ ✩ ✩
Cleanliness: ✩ ✩ ✩ ✩ ✩
Insect Control: ✩ ✩

KEY INFORMATION

ADDRESS: Marys Peak
Campground
c/o Waldport
Ranger District
1130 Forestry Lane
Waldport, OR
97394

OPERATED BY: Siuslaw National
Forest

INFORMATION: (541) 563-3211

OPEN: Campground is
open from April
until whenever
the road closes,
which is based on
snow but is no
later than Decem-
ber 1; after Sep-
tember 30, there is
no water and no
services in the
campground

SITES: 6

EACH SITE: Picnic table, fire
pit, shade trees

ASSIGNMENT: First come,
first served; no
reservations

REGISTRATION: Self-registration
on site

FACILITIES: Vault toilets

PARKING: At campsites

FEE: $10; $10 per
additional vehicle

ELEVATION: 4,097 feet

RESTRICTIONS: *Pets:* On leash only
Fires: In fire pits
only
Alcohol: Permitted
Vehicles: No RVs or
trailers

country skiers. The campground is closed from December 1 to March 31, but a Northwest Forest Pass buys you the privilege to park near Connor's Camp and enjoy as much nonmotorized recreation as you can cram into a short winter day.

The same meadows that are cross-country routes in winter are flower-filled delights in the spring. Predominant year-round are the evergreens: Douglas, noble, and Pacific silver fir at the higher elevations, with an understory of sword ferns, salal, and oxalis. Stands of western hemlock grow so thickly at lower elevations that the lack of sunshine keeps the underbrush at a low ebb. To help visitors get optimum enjoyment out of the abundant foliage, a quintet of hiking trails offer various rambles around the knobby presence of Marys Peak. They range from the easy, looped Meadowedge Trail that leaves from the campground and to the top of Marys Peak to the moderate 2.4-mile East Ridge Trail through stands of old-growth Douglas fir and Sitka spruce forest to the lengthier North Ridge Trail (5.5 miles) that links Marys Peak with Woods Creek Road down. All in all, 12 miles of trails will take you through two vegetation zones, past old-growth noble fir stands, along the same route once used by sheepherders, and when conditions are right, amongst some of the best wildflower displays in the Coast Range.

Not all flora has enjoyed an untrammeled existence on Marys Peak, however. In the past, the Forest Service allowed disastrous quantities of timber (particularly noble fir) to be cut. A renewed effort is underway to reforest these areas, and Marys Peak Scenic Botanical Area is an experiment to preserve the noble fir and to restimulate its growth. This will not only restore the natural beauty of the area, but also continue to provide habitat for woodland creatures such as deer, grouse, and squirrels.

Sidetrips in the Marys Peak vicinity include the South Fork Alsea River Byway, the Benton County Scenic Loop, William L. Finley National Wildlife Refuge, the Willamette Floodplain, Benton County Historical Museum in Philomath, Corvallis Arts Center, and Horner Museum (also in Corvallis). There's a nice bike path between Corvallis and Philomath that follows

MAP

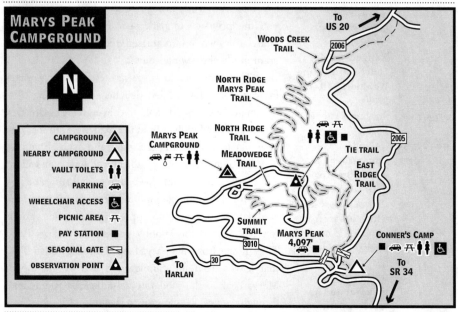

MARYS PEAK CAMPGROUND

N

Legend	
CAMPGROUND	▲
NEARBY CAMPGROUND	△
VAULT TOILETS	⚤
PARKING	🚐
WHEELCHAIR ACCESS	♿
PICNIC AREA	⛱
PAY STATION	■
SEASONAL GATE	⤫
OBSERVATION POINT	▲

To US 20

WOODS CREEK TRAIL

2006

NORTH RIDGE MARYS PEAK TRAIL

NORTH RIDGE TRAIL

2005

MARYS PEAK CAMPGROUND

MEADOWEDGE TRAIL

TIE TRAIL

EAST RIDGE TRAIL

SUMMIT TRAIL

MARYS PEAK 4,097'

3010

CONNER'S CAMP

30

To HARLAN

To SR 34

the Willamette and Marys Rivers. Mountain biking on the zillion forest roads in Siuslaw National Forest requires a very good map.

GETTING THERE

To reach Marys Peak from Philomath (6 miles southwest of Corvallis), follow Alsea Highway (SR 34) southwest roughly 10 miles to Marys Peak Road (FS 30) and turn right. Follow Marys Peak Road, which becomes FS 3010, to its end and the campground.

GPS COORDINATES

UTM Zone (WGS84)	10T
Easting	0456041
Northing	4928047
Latitude	N 44.5044°
Longitude	W 123.553°

APPENDIX A: CAMPING EQUIPMENT CHECKLIST

Except for the large and bulky items on this list, I keep a plastic storage container full of the essentials for car camping so they're ready to go when I am. I make a last-minute check of the inventory, resupply anything that's low or missing, and away I go.

COOKING UTENSILS

Bottle opener

Bottles of salt, pepper, spices, sugar, cooking oil, and maple syrup in water-proof, spillproof containers

Can opener

Corkscrew

Cups, plastic or tin

Dish soap (biodegradable), sponge, and towel

Flatware

Food of your choice

Frying pan, spatula

Fuel for stove

Lighter, matches in waterproof container

Plates

Pocketknife

Fire starter

Pot with lid

Stove

Tin foil

Wooden spoon

FIRST-AID KIT

Aspirin

Band-Aids

First-aid cream

Gauze pads

Insect repellent

Moleskin

Sunscreen, lip balm

Tape, waterproof adhesive

SLEEPING GEAR

Pillow

Sleeping bag

Sleeping pad, inflatable or insulated

Tent with ground tarp and rainfly

MISCELLANEOUS

Bath soap (biodegradable), washcloth, and towel

Camp chair

Candles

Cooler

Deck of cards

Flashlight/headlamp

Paper towels

Plastic zip-top bags

Sunglasses

Toilet paper

Water bottle

Wool blanket

OPTIONAL

Barbecue grill

Binoculars

Field guides on bird, plant, and wildlife identification

Fishing rod and tackle

Lantern

Maps (road, trail, topographic, etc.)

APPENDIX B: SOURCES OF INFORMATION

AAA AUTOMOBILE CLUB OF OREGON
600 SW Market
Portland, OR 97201
(503) 222-6700
www.aaa.com

BUREAU OF LAND MANAGEMENT
P.O. Box 2965, Portland, OR 97232
1515 SW 5th Avenue, Portland, OR 97201
(503) 952-6001
www.or.blm.gov

CRATER LAKE NATIONAL PARK (NPS)
P.O. Box 7, Crater Lake, OR 97604
(541) 594-2211
www.nps.gov/crla

HELLS CANYON NATIONAL RECREATION AREA (USFS)
P.O. Box 490, Enterprise, OR 97828
(541) 426-4978
www.fs.fed.us/hellscanyon/

THE MAZAMAS (HIKING AND CLIMBING CLUB)
909 NW 19th Street, Portland, OR 97209
(503) 227-2345
www.mazamas.org

NATURE OF THE NORTHWEST (MAPS AND FIELD GUIDES)
800 NE Oregon, #5, Portland, OR 97232
(503) 731-4444
www.naturenw.org

OREGON COAST VISITORS ASSOCIATION
P.O. Box 670, Newport, OR 97365
(541) 574-2679 or (888) 628-2101
www.oregon-coast.org

OREGON DEPARTMENT OF FISH AND WILDLIFE
P.O. Box 59, Portland, OR 97207
(503) 229-5410
www.dfw.state.or.us

OREGON TOURISM COMMISSION
775 Summer Street NE, Salem, OR 97310
(800) 547-7842 (toll free nationwide)
www.traveloregon.com

OREGON STATE PARKS AND RECREATION
1115 Commercial Street NE
Salem, OR 97301
(503) 378-8605
www.prd.state.or.us

OUTDOOR RECREATION INFORMATION CENTER (NPS AND USFS INFO FOR THE NORTHWEST)
222 Yale North (inside REI)
Seattle, WA 98109-5429
(206) 220-7450
www.nps.gov/ccso/oric.htm

RESERVATIONS NORTHWEST
P.O. Box 500, Portland, OR 97207-0500
(503) 731-3411 or (800) 452-5687
www.prd.state.or.us/reservation.html

U.S. FISH AND WILDLIFE SERVICE (OREGON OFFICE)
P.O. Box 111, Lakeview, OR 97630
(541) 947-3315
www.fws.gov/oregonfwo/

U.S. FOREST SERVICE (PACIFIC NORTH-WEST REGIONAL HEADQUARTERS)
P.O. Box 3623, Portland, OR 97208
333 SW 1st Avenue, Portland, OR 97204
(503) 221-2877
www.fs.fed.us/r6

INDEX

**THE BEST
IN TENT
CAMPING
OREGON**

ABOUT THE AUTHORS

JEANNE LOUISE PYLE is a transplanted Marylander who has lived in the Pacific Northwest for 30 years. Her love of the outdoors led to authoring the first book of *The Best in Tent Camping* series in 1994. Pyle currently resides in Bellingham, Washington.

PAUL GERALD is a professional freelance writer and lover of the outdoors whose work has appeared in newspapers around the country, as well as *Northwest Airlines WorldTraveler, Dish Magazine, Weissmann Travel Reports,* and Nike's web site. Gerald is also the author of *60 Hikes within 60 Miles: Portland, Day & Overnight Hikes: Oregon's Pacific Crest Trail* (both publshed by Menasha Ridge Press), and *Breakfast in Bridgetown: The Definitive Guide to Portland's Favorite Meal.*